All About Muscle

A User's Guide

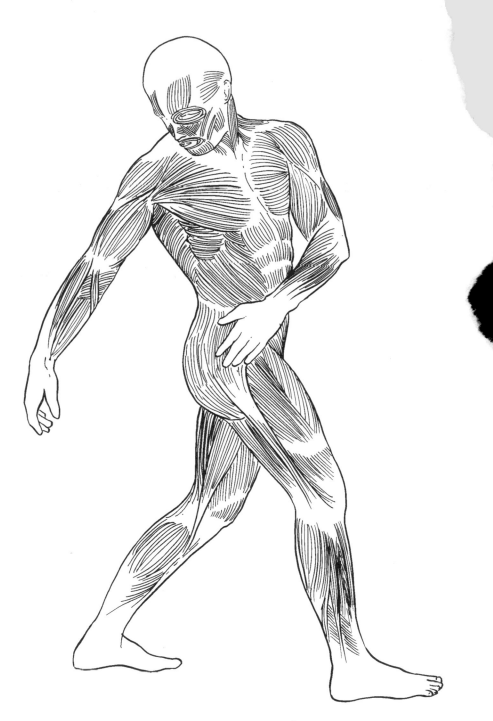

FRONTSIPIECE   Glorify God in your body. I *Corinthians*, 6:20.

All About Muscle

A User's Guide

Irwin M. Siegel, M.D.

Demos

New York

Demos Medical Publishing, Inc., 386 Park Avenue South,
New York, New York 10016

Library of Congress Cataloging-in-Publication Data

Siegel, Irwin M., 1927–
    All about muscle : a user's guide / Irwin M. Siegel.
      p.   cm.
    Includes bibliographical references and index.
    ISBN 1–888799–42–0
    1. Muscles—Popular works.   I. Title.
QP321.S44   2000
616.7′4—dc21   00-035860

Printed in the United States of America

Acknowledgments

The author acknowledges the following people for their assistance in the preparation of this book.

Mrs. Jackie Abern for her patient transcription and reworking of the manuscript.

Ms. Patricia Casey for expert proofing of the manuscript and critical comments.

Artists Kurt Peterson and Kristen Wienandt for their outstanding illustrations.

Syed Maghrabi for bibliographic assistance.

The clinic staff of the Muscle Disease Clinics of the Rush-Presbyterian–St.Luke's Medical Center, Bridget Carey (MDA program services coordinator) and Karen Boone (secretary), and the Evanston Hospital, particularly Rita Yager (nurse), for their able help with the multidisciplinary management of our patient roster.

Chris Galietta and Mike Fitzhenry, seating consultants at Metro Rehab, Worth, Illinois, for keeping our patients comfortable and functional in their wheelchairs and for keeping me up to date on the latest in mobility technology.

Orthotists Gene Bernardini and his able staff at the Ballert Orthotic Laboratory, Chicago, Illinois, and Ron Grimaud, Scheck & Siress, Inc., Chicago, Illinois, for assistance in the area of their expertise.

My able colleagues, Drs. Matthew Meriggioli, Julie Rowin, Robert Wright, Peter Heydemann, Larry Bernstein, Nicholas Vick, Christopher Goetz, and the late Dr. Harold L. Klawans, for continuing tuition in the fascinating fields of myology, neuromuscular disease, and allied neurologic conditions.

The Muscular Dystrophy Association, particularly Mr. Robert Ross, Senior Vice President and Executive Director, and Margaret Wahl, R.N., B.S.N., Senior Medical and Science Writer, for their encouragement and assistance.

Demos Medical Publishing, Inc., of New York, especially Diana M. Schneider, Ph.D., Publisher, and Joan Wolk, Managing Editor, for patiently and skillfully shepherding the book through editing and publication.

"Guerir quelquefois, soulanger souvent,
consoler toujours."
To cure sometimes, to relieve often,
to comfort always.
Folk saying (French, 15th century)

This book is dedicated to my patients.

Contents

Foreword

Irwin Siegel has once again come up with a remarkably informative and readable book, straddling the bridge between the academic and clinical on the one hand and the intelligent lay reader on the other. Aptly titled *All About Muscle,* the text provides a bird's-eye view of all aspects of muscle function and dysfunction and intermittently also probes the depths to further stimulate the interest of the reader.

It comprehensively covers the basic structure and function of normal muscle, from the anatomic, physiologic, and biochemical aspects, as well as some of the common disorders of muscle such, as the muscular dystrophies, and of the motor nerves that control the muscle, such as amyotrophic lateral sclerosis (ALS, or Lou Gehrig's disease).

Having devoted his professional life to the practice of orthopaedic surgery, Irwin Siegel has always had a much broader canvas, including the management and rehabilitation of children with muscular dystrophy, about which he has written extensively. He has also shown a remarkable insight into communication and rapport directly with the children themselves. Every now and again the neuroscientist in him has also come to the surface asking questions about mechanisms and pathogenesis of disorder. This book also contains ample advice to the able-bodied for improving their muscle function through appropriate exercise.

Added to this remarkable mixture of different aspects of muscle, there are interesting vignettes and quotations from the historical literature, vividly illustrated by some of the classical images in the field. Finally, for quick reference is a useful glossary of commonly used medical and scientific terms, often taken for granted by the professionals but totally incomprehensible to the lay person.

This book should attract a wide range of interest and, given its clarity of content and lucidity of style, it should readily achieve a combined role of both educating and entertaining the reader.

Victor Dubowitz
Emeritus Professor of Paediatrics
Imperial College School of Science and Medicine
Hammersmith Campus
London

Preface

Everything expresses itself in movement, and the ability to move is one of the qualities that defines life. I have always been interested in movement and fascinated by the speed, power, and grace with which muscular action enlivens our bodies. Perhaps that is why I chose orthopaedic surgery as my medical specialty—to study at close hand the musculoskeletal system in order to better understand how normal muscle functions, and through such knowledge to search for and remedy the causes of muscular dysfunction and disease.

In addition to a general practice of orthopaedics, which includes the diagnosis and treatment of injuries, congenital malformations, tumors, degenerative diseases, deficiency states, and infections of muscle, I have for the past 39 years directed muscle disease clinics for the Muscular Dystrophy Association of America. Through my work with the Association, I have had the opportunity to diagnose and treat almost every variety of muscle disease in children and adults. Over 100 research papers and two books (*The Clinical Management of Muscle Disease*, J.B. Lippincott, 1977, and *Muscle and Its Diseases*, Yearbook Medical Publishers, 1986) were borne of this work. In thinking of these matters and in counseling patients and their families over the years, it seemed to me that the larger public would want to be informed and enlightened about the organ system that motivates their every move and the largest tissue mass their body carries. I had similar motives in writing my previous book, *All About Bone* (Demos, 1998), which deals with the skeletal system in a similar way.

Thus, *All About Muscle* came to be. This amazing and elegant tissue interfaces with, affects, and is affected by almost every other organ in the body. In considering muscle, we also have to take a look at such things as circulation, nutrition, bones and joints of course, the nervous system by all means, and so forth.

We start with a quick overview to whet the reader's appetite and then a brief bit of history for those so inclined. We then proceed to a concise outline of basic science (anatomy, histology, chemistry)—just enough for the intelligent reader to make sense of the chapters that follow. Then we apply our newly acquired fundamental knowledge to practical matters such as exercise, diet, muscle building, relaxation, and the disorders and injuries of muscle.

Ludwig Wittgenstein (1889–1951) once said, "Whatever can be said at all can be said clearly, and whatever cannot be said clearly should not be said at all." I have attempted to follow this principle in writing this book, and I hope I have been successful in collating a vast amount of technical material into understandable text and providing sound practical advice when it comes to matters of medical interest.

Although love makes the world go round, muscle gives it the push. If you are at all interested in how it goes about this, read on.

Irwin M. Siegel, M.D.
Evanston, Illinois
January 2000

Introduction

Muscle: From the Greek, *a mouse.* Probably so named because of its quick movements and the similarity of its tendon to a mouse's tail.

Consider muscle. It is the body's largest tissue. You have about 650 muscles (more than 50 in your face alone), and they account for 35 percent of body weight in women and 45 percent in men. Contrast this with bone, which makes up only 12 percent of your body weight. The bones of someone weighing 110 pounds weigh only 13 pounds. You have more than 30 muscles in each forearm and hand, and you use over 200 different muscles when you walk. With the help of electrical input from the nervous system, muscle converts chemical energy to mechanical work while it gives off heat—and it does this silently. Furthermore, its job is accomplished at approximately the proficiency of a diesel engine, 40 percent, which beats the internal combustion motor of your automobile, operating at only 8 percent to 10 percent efficiency. Muscle can be switched on within a thousandth of a second and can accelerate from 0 to 90 mph in 30 seconds. It is versatile enough to use both carbohydrates and fats as fuel. Like a computer, it has a built-in servomechanism (feedback control). And, lest we forget, it is good to eat!

The dictionary defines muscle as a contractile tissue, found in animals, the function of which is to produce motion, but it gives no hint as to the exquisite elegance of this versatile substance. All our motions are powered by muscles that act through the leverage systems that our joints provide. (Even the wheel is a set of levers disguised as spokes, working in sequence to provide circular motion.) Movement is a vital and necessary life force, and the history of science has in great part been based on the investigation of why and how things move. Our language incorporates movement metaphor. We drag our feet, jump to conclusions, wrestle with problems, and grasp answers. Our emotional state is often described as uptight, stiff-necked, tense, rigid, or slack, or in musical expressions such as "keyed up" or "highly strung."

Muscle is central to our evolution as human beings. It raised us from the four-legged position so we could survey the savanna to uncover predators and seek out food. It enabled us to fully straighten our knees. Apes cannot do this; they lack the necessary inside knee muscle and must walk in a crouched position. Spiders, on the other hand, have muscles to bend the knees but none to straighten them—to do this, fluid must be pumped in, in the same way that turning on the water straightens a garden hose. If a spider becomes too dry, it cannot straighten its legs.

Muscle provides us with superbly versatile manipulative tools in the structure of our hands, distinguishing us from lower primate forms through, among other features, thumbs that can oppose to better grasp, pinch, and perform manipulative tasks. It can load our molars with a force of 150 pounds—more than enough to chomp away at the toughest steak.

Muscles enable the impala to jump as far as 25 feet and the cheetah to achieve speeds close to 70 miles an hour during its chase. Muscles empower a 300-pound ostrich to outrun every other two-legged animal at 30 miles per hour. The male toadfish calls his mate by contracting the muscles surrounding his gas-filled swim bladder at the amazing rate of 200 times per second. Diamondback rattlesnakes can rattle their tails 90 times per second.

Muscles make it possible for camels to raise and advance both legs on one side at one time and for horses to run with all four hooves in the air at once. Muscles endow the remarkable trapdoor spider with the strength to hold the door to its nest closed with a force of 14 ounces, some 140 times its weight of 0.1 ounce, which is equivalent to a 150-pound man pulling with a force of 10 tons. Muscles empower our eyes to move some 100,000 times every day (to exercise our legs this much we would have to walk at least 50 miles). And, no matter whether they are lifting, throwing, pushing, pulling, running, or stooping, muscles do all of this by shortening (contracting).

An incredible 100,000 muscles power an elephant's trunk, the most supple and versatile appendage in all of nature. Among other things, this nose tipped with a lip allows the elephant to feel below to see where he is going. An elephant's hind feet always step where his front feet have been, but because elephants are so large that they cannot look down, the trunk is often used to feel the ground just ahead and underneath their massive heads.

A snake is essentially two long tubes of muscle. Inside is the digestive tract, pushing food along by waves of contraction called peristalsis. Outside is the body wall. A snake slithers forward by bending his body in an S-shaped curve from side to side.

Like other body tissues, muscle has a circadian rhythm. That is to say, its contraction strength varies with the time of day. The hand grip is strongest around 6 P.M. and weakest at about 3 A.M..

Strange as it may seem, muscles generate sound as they contract and relax, which they do continually when we are awake. If you doubt this, put both thumbs gently in your ears and make a fist. The low rumble you hear is the sound made by the contraction of the muscles of your forearm and the tighter you make a fist, the louder the sound becomes. Our ears are insensitive to the 25 Hertz (cycles per second) low-frequency sound of muscle so we ordinarily do not hear it contracting. However, it can be picked up by a stethoscope applied over a contracting muscle. Also, by placing your index finger next to your partially closed eye, you will feel a vibration due to muscle contraction. The study of muscle sound could lead to better understanding of muscle physiology and pathology (including the heart muscle) and even of certain types of animal communication.

Muscles come in all sizes. The tiniest muscle in the body is the stapedius, measuring 1/20 of an inch, which activates the inner ear. This is the muscle that is overworked at a rock concert due to noise. Chronic fatigue with damage of the stapedius can lead to permanent hearing loss. The smallest "voluntary" muscle is the levator palpebrae superior, which raises the upper eyelid. Our largest muscle is the quadriceps, which straightens the knee. In women, however, one muscle shows an extraordinary increase in size. During pregnancy, the womb (uterus), which is composed of smooth muscle, increases in weight from just over an ounce to more than two pounds—some thirty times larger! Our longest muscle, the sartorius, extends from the waist to the knee, and is so named because tailors used to work sitting cross-legged on the floor, stretching this muscle. The muscle claiming the greatest area is the latissimus dorsi, the flat muscle of the back. Our strongest muscle is the one we sit on, the gluteus maximus. Ounce for ounce, however, the strongest muscles in our body are the masseters, located on each side of the jaw. Working together, the masseters generate a biting force of approximately 150 pounds. Our fastest muscles are those of our eyes, which contract in less than 1/100 of a second. By contrast, our slowest muscle is the soleus in the lower leg, which helps keep the body upright by contracting in 1/10 of a second.

There actually are three kinds of muscles. One class of muscle is called *voluntary* or *striated* muscle. As its name implies, it includes all the muscles we use when we move consciously. Some striated muscles, however, such as those involved in breathing, are both voluntary and involuntary in their use. That is, respiration can be controlled by will to a certain extent, but it ordinarily goes on without conscious effort on our part.

Involuntary or *smooth* muscle includes *multiunit* and *visceral* muscle. Multiunit smooth muscle is made of independent fibers that are separated from each other but linked by a single nerve ending. This type of muscle is found around blood vessels. It shapes the lens of the eye and makes the hair stand on end with goose bumps when we are frightened or cold. *Erector pili,* tiny muscles in the skin, cause the hair to rise. This can make an animal appear larger and more fierce. It also provides insulation by raising the skin at the base of the hair and closing the pores, conserving heat. All of this occurs as a reflex response. Most smooth muscle, however, is visceral. It surrounds nearly all of the body's organs, and the muscle cells are connected by junctions known as *nexi*. These connections permit the cells to communicate and perform as a single unit. Smooth muscle is distinguished by its slow contraction and relaxation periods and its rhythmic action.

Finally, there is *heart* muscle, which is built like voluntary muscle but acts like smooth muscle. Cardiac muscle has the potential to contract spontaneously and carries electrical impulses that originate in areas of the heart known as pacemakers. Cardiac muscle cells are unified by function, and thus the heart beats. In fact, due to the unique electrical properties of its cells, the heart will keep on beating temporarily when removed from the body. Even small bits of cardiac muscle will continue to pulse if they are kept in warm salt water.

It has been a long road to our present knowledge of muscle. There have been some interesting sights and amazing insights along the way. Let's take a look at what has come before.

1

A Short Biography of Muscle

"Citius, altius, fortius."

— Latin motto for the Olympic games: "Swifter, higher, stronger."

Muscular strength and agility have been written about since the beginnings of recorded history. The ancient Greeks sought their ideals in games. Herodotus relates that Xerxes, the king of Persia, preparing to wage war on the Greeks in 480 B.C., found his enemy engaged in the games at Olympia. In the ninth century B.C.., Homer in his epics noted that games were common pastimes among heroic warriors. To honor their gods and display their muscular physiques, Greeks trained and competed naked. The Greek word *gymnasium* means a place where one exercises in the nude. To the Greek mind, shame of nudity was the mark of a barbarian.

The Romans were an active, martial people. They considered exercise and recreation desirable but they despised Greek athletics. Roman games were not contests but spectacles and circuses. Combat between gladiators and fights with beasts soaked the sand of the Roman coliseums with blood.

The misplaced piety and harsh asceticism of the medieval church drew a solemn veil over an earthy and robust time. By the sixth century, Christian emperors had put an end to athletic festivals and other spectacles. Originating somewhat before the eleventh century, tournaments with mounted knights captured the fancy of the nobility. Commoners were left with less romantic pursuits that included football, bowling, wrestling, and hockey. Edward III, preparing England for war with France, forbade all athletics save archery, which was always a popular pastime among the English and served the king well in time of national conflict. Dancing was, of course, condemned by the clergy because of its association with festivals having pagan rites and its sometimes flaunting of sexual license.

Protestant reformers challenged the benefits of organized games and exercise, especially on the Sabbath. Although religious enthusiasm restrained popular entertainments and games, exercise began again to win favor during the enlightenment of the eighteenth century. Proselytized by Rousseau and organized in such central European countries as Germany and Scandinavia (Denmark became the first country to introduce compulsory physical education in its schools), gymnastics came to be regarded as an important part of education.

However, it was the Victorians who took the ball and ran with it (no pun intended). In fact, one of the great Victorian philosophers, Herbert Spencer, even held that, "All breaches of the law of health are physical sins." During Victorian times there was a surge of interest in fitness, and the Latin ideal espoused by Juvenal of *mens sane in corpore sano* (a fit mind in a fit body) was their maxim for healthy living.

The health-conscious Victorians invented athletics. The term *calisthenics* was coined in 1859. It meant "beautiful strength." Sport was also associated with Christian virtue and was described in phrases such as "it's not cricket" and "fair play." Sport was considered a test of moral strength made all the more admirable through its qualities of courage and stamina. The Victorians also developed quaint methods to encourage proper posture, particularly in young women (Figure 1-1).

In seeking to expand the power of our muscles, we mastered mechanical energy. Just as machinery was devised from the application of muscular power, the principles of mechanics offered instruction in the way muscles work. The study of body movement (biomechanics-kinesiology) is based on mechanical principles. Although he performed no experiments, Aristotle (384–322 B.C.) expostulated the fundamental principles of animal motion 24 centuries ago. He determined laws of movement by describing the action of limbs and then analyzing the motion on geometric principles. Aristotle was the first to understand that an animal must shift its weight about its center of

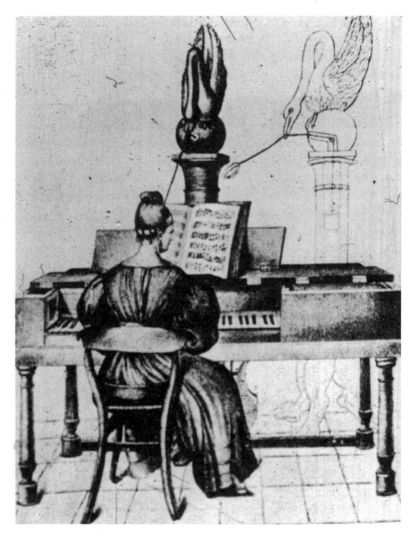

FIGURE 1-1 Victorian apparatus for encouraging proper posture in the well-bred young woman.

gravity in order to walk erect. However, he also thought the function of the brain was to cool the heart!

Galen explored the positions and actions of muscles 500 years later. He described how muscles worked in opposing pairs—agonist and antagonist. He was the first to distinguish between motor and sensory nerves, and the first to realize that muscles act by contracting. Galen believed that "animal spirits" coursing along the motor nerves caused muscles to contract.

Human dissection was forbidden by the church during the Dark Ages (476–1000 A.D.), and it was not until the fifteenth century that the study of motion itself began to move.

Leonardo da Vinci (1452–1519) wrote that "motion is the cause of all life." He was an ingenious engineer who tested mechanical principles with structures of his own design, studying anatomy and physiology and applying them in his exacting art. Leonardo distinguished many different muscles by their size, shape, and movement. He realized that a muscle moves solely in response to the nerve from which it receives a stimulus. Leonardo's models included cords representing muscles attached to a skeleton. He saw that if one of a pair shortened, its partner lengthened. In detailed drawings, this genius illustrated how the configuration of muscles change as they move our limbs. He once set out to discover the exact physical location of the soul, reasoning that it "must be at the center of the brain, for judgment apparently resides in the place where all the senses meet, and where imagination, intellect and common sense live." The eminent Flemish anatomist and physician Andreas Vesalius (1514–1564) illustrated the anatomy of muscle from his own dissections in his monumental work, *De Humani Corpus Fabrica Libri Septem* (seven books on the structure of the human body), said to be "one of the most noble and magnificent volumes in the history of printing."

The scientific revolution heralded by the Polish astronomer Nicholas Copernicus's (1473–1543) description of the revolution of the heavenly spheres established principles and methods that also accounted for the movements of human beings. Galileo (1564–1642) applied mathematics to physical movement, using measurable phenomena, such as mass, acceleration, weight, space, velocity, and time, to mark the beginning of classical mechanics. Lacking a proper clock, he often took his pulse to time his experiments!

One of Galileo's pupils, Alfonso Borelli, turned his attention to the human body. In his book on the motion of animals, which was published in 1630, he depicted animals as machines moved by levers powered by muscles. Borelli sought to measure forces generated by different muscles but, like Galen before him, he believed that the flow of "animal spirits" stimulated by the brain caused their contraction. Borelli believed that these spirits filled the pores in muscles with an unknown substance, causing a fermentation-like reaction that stimulated shortening. This theory was challenged by Francis Glisson, an English physician who is best known for his work on rickets. Glisson showed that muscle fibers contracted when stimulated.

In 1700 the Italian Georgio Baglivi characterized smooth muscle, distinguishing it from its striated cousin. The Danish anatomist Nicolaus Steno described the heart as a muscle. It was becoming apparent that the nervous system exercised different controls over different kinds of muscle. During the late eighteenth century Luigi Galvani noted that the muscles of a dissected frog contracted when touched with a scalpel. He deduced that nerve conducted an electrical current to muscle. Thus electricity took the place of animal spirits as the stimulation for muscular contraction. In the next century the use of electricity in the treatment of disease was pioneered by Guillaume Duchenne (Figure 1-2).

The quantum leap in the study of muscle and movement was made by Edward Muybridge, a pioneering photographer who first photographed animals and human beings in motion. In 1887 he published some 4,700 images under the title *The Human Figure in Motion,* with almost as many of animals in action. Muybridge tracked movement at 1/6000th of a second, documenting the subtle details of the body in motion. With the advent of motion pictures, the structure of movement could be further caught, frozen, and studied.

Meanwhile, knowledge of just how muscles generate motion was growing. In America Henry Pickering Bowditch proposed the "all-or-none" principle of muscular contraction. This principle states that an individual muscle fiber contracts completely or not at all, and that the strength of the stimulus determines the *number* of fibers called upon to contract. Charles Sherington published *The Integrative Action of the Nervous System* in 1906. This was a turning point in our understanding of the principles of *kinesiology* (the study of mechanics and anatomy in relation to human movement). Sherington first described the principle of *reciprocal innervation,* in which nerve impulses stimulating a particular muscle at the same time inhibit the nerves of its antagonist, ensuring the harmonious working of groups of muscles through a so-called "muscular sense" capable of appreciating mechanical tension and mediated by microscopic spindle-shaped tensors embedded in the muscles and linked to

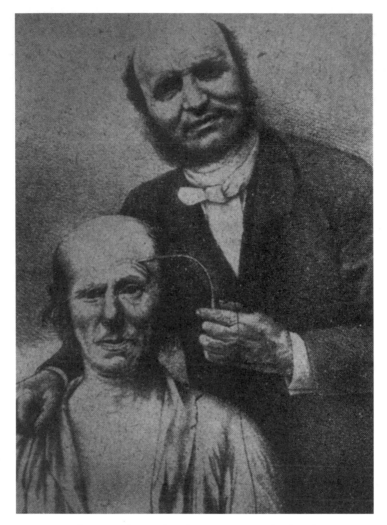

FIGURE 1-2   Duchenne inducing faradic stimulation of a facial muscle.

the spinal cord by nerve fibers entering through the sensory roots. Sherington won a Nobel Prize in physiology for his work.

Descartes (1596–1650) had thought that muscular contraction was generated by animal spirits propelled by the brain through tubelike nerves. He also believed that the pincal gland—the only unpaired structure in the brain that sits in its exact center—was the seat of the soul. Modern investigators continued to elucidate the structure and chemistry of muscle. Among them was A. V. Hill, who was awarded a Nobel prize in

1992 for his experiments on the physiology of muscle contraction, which included his concept of an "oxygen debt," the ability of muscle to recharge after exercise through the use of oxygen. Hugh Huxley of Massachusetts and Andrew Huxley of England—not related and working independently—simultaneously described the mechanism by which muscle contracts. The research of Albert Szent-Gyorgi investigated the chemical nature of muscles, while others worked to describe its energy metabolism.

At the same time as the basic science of muscle was being investigated, clinicians such as Duchenne, Gowers, and Meryon were characterizing its diseases. Nicolas Andry (1658–1747) had already laid the groundwork for rational clinical management. Andry coined the word *orthopaedics* from the Greek *ortho* = straight and *pais* = child. He founded the specialty but did not publish until he was in his eighties. Andry postulated that muscles were the primary instruments in shaping a child's body and advocated playing on these instruments to correct orthopaedic deformity. Along these same lines, another French physician, Jacques Delpech (b. 1777), was the first to section tendons to treat deformity due to contracture.

The explosion of medical technology after World War II, particularly in the fields of electrophysiology, microscopy, physical chemistry, and molecular biology, led to an exponential growth in our understanding of muscle and its disorders. Before we consider pathology, however, let's see how normal muscle works.

2

Muscle, By and Large

"The skillful man is within the function of his skill, a different integration, a different nervous and muscular and psychological organization . . ."

Bernard DeVoto (Across the Wide Missouri, 1947)

All animal movement is the work of muscle. Muscles work by *contracting*—that is to say, they *always* pull, *never* push. Even if you push in a door, every muscle cell involved in this task is at work pulling! The body is engineered to convert this pulling into pushing.

SIZE

The number of muscle fibers in your body is determined at birth. In this respect, muscle is similar to nervous tissue. The number of fibers does not multiply, but individual fibers do enlarge with work. This accounts for the size and strength of the muscles of a weight lifter contrasted with those of an inactive desk clerk, even though their muscles contain the same number of fibers. Isaac Nesson developed the largest biceps ever recorded—it had a diameter of 26 1/8 inches. Theoretically, the maximum energy output of a man is approximately 6 hp. The highest recorded output to date is 4.5 hp; 0.5 hp can be sustained almost indefinitely.

Muscle fibers can be short or long, but their diameter is always less than their length (most fibers measure from 0.01 mm to 0.1 mm across). Many individual fibers make up each muscle. There are approximately 650 skeletal muscles in the body (about three times as many muscles as bones), containing about 250,000,000 striated muscle fibers. In the eye these fibers have a diameter of 20 microns (one micron is one millionth of a meter). The fibers of the limbs range in size from 10 to 100 microns, being largest in male athletes.

Each muscle obeys the same "all-or-none" principle as the nerve fiber that controls it—either it contracts or it doesn't. Muscle works by converting chemical energy to mechanical energy. Less than half of the potential energy available is converted, and the remainder is lost as heat. This is why your body temperature rises when you perform strenuous work. Even at rest, the heat produced during the relatively efficient conversion of chemical to mechanical energy in muscle maintains body temperature in animals exposed to the cold. The muscular movements associated with shivering liberate heat so it is not wasted, as it is in most man-made machines. Sometimes enough heat is produced to boil a quart of water. Shivering may be better than a heating pad or exercise when it comes to warming the body. In some cases of modest hypothermia, heat from an external source may actually be counterproductive because it inhibits the shivering response.

Timing

There is no uniformity concerning the total time taken for a contraction or the interval between regular muscle contractions. Take heartbeat as an example. An elephant's heart contracts every 2.5 seconds, whereas a canary's heart contracts approximately 17 times *each* second. As everyone has experienced, the human heart can change from a 60/minute resting pace to as much as three times that rate during vigorous exercise.

Even a fast heartbeat is not the fastest muscular rhythm available to the body. Finger-tapping can be speedier for a time. Human beings are outclassed in this endeavor by the wing beats of many insects. The wings of bees vibrate at 250 cycles per second, and those of mosquitoes vibrate up to 585 cycles. All this is possible because these insect wing muscles do not abide by the conventional relationship between nerve and muscle. A voluntary muscle twitches only once in response to a single nerve impulse, whereas the remarkably high-speed muscle of the insect wing twitches many times in reaction to each stimulus.

Such wing muscles do not normally relax after contracting. This allows the wing muscle of some insects to generate more energy than any other animal tissue. Other cells move, but only muscle cells moves by contraction. An amoeba slides about, white blood cells glide as they stalk invading bacteria, and the whiplike tail of a sperm cell lashes to propel it. All of these movements are controlled by two special proteins, *actin* and *myosin* (see Chapter 6).

MUSCLE TYPES

As mentioned previously, there are three distinct types of muscle, each of which performs a specific task (Figure 2-1). These three types of muscle are composed of different kinds of muscle cells. *Skeletal* muscle cells are the longest and have multiple nuclei. *Cardiac* and *smooth* muscle cells have only a single nucleus. *Skeletal* (striated) muscle carries out voluntary movements such as walking. Because these muscles must counteract gravity, they must stay alert to prevent the body from falling. *Tone* is the term used to describe this state of readiness. Without tone we would all look like rag dolls.

   Cardiac muscle keeps the heart pumping. Cardiac muscle cells connect with each other through junctions called *intercalated disks*. This allows them to pass electrical signals from the heart's natural pacemaker (the sinoatrial node) throughout the heart so that it can continue its harmonious pumping action. Not much bigger than a clenched fist, the heart contracts and expands 70 times each minute in a man, 78 times in a woman,

FIGURE 2-1   The three kinds of muscle cells.

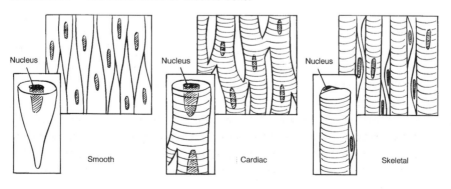

Nucleus · Smooth · Nucleus · Cardiac · Nucleus · Skeletal

130 times in an infant, and 90 times in a 12-year-old. Your heart pumps up to 1,500 gallons of blood a day. In your lifetime this would fill 13 supertankers containing one million barrels each! The heart directs this volume to the 60,000 miles of circulatory conduits. The heart pumps more blood when the body is horizontal because it is less impeded by gravity. A swimmer's heart can pump up to 20 percent more blood because he or she is essentially weightless in the water.

The slender cylindrical fibers of *smooth* muscle are arranged in sheets around blood vessels and internal organs. Most smooth muscle is *visceral,* surrounding nearly all of the body's major organs. Some smooth muscle is made of independent fibers. These so-called *multiunit* fibers seldom contract spontaneously. An example is the piloerector muscle attached to the base of each hair follicle. These tiny muscles pull the hair erect, causing "goose bumps," and bristle a cat's fur when it is frightened. Smooth muscle has the slowest contraction and relaxation periods of any muscle, and its action is quite rhythmic. Smooth muscle is able to maintain its tension despite varying degrees of stretching. Although controlled by nerves, smooth muscle also can be activated by stretch. This is how the bladder, when full, automatically begins to contract. It also is why we get a "lump" in our throat when we are sad and about to cry. The normal peristaltic wave that moves smoothly to our stomach is reversed, causing a feeling like a knot or lump in the throat, which makes it difficult to swallow.

FUNCTION

The size of the pupil in the front of the eyes is modulated by the *sphincter* and *dilator* muscles of the iris, the colored part surrounding the pupil. Pupils respond to dim light by dilating and to bright light by contracting, to keep light from damaging the eye. They respond to emotion in a similar fashion. Fear or excitement enlarges the pupils. This probably is due to the brain's need to see more of what is happening in a potentially dangerous situation. On the other hand, unpleasant scenes that do not evoke anxiety cause the pupils to constrict. Pupil reaction may reflect the level of the viewer's interest. Men's pupils dilate when viewing pictures of nude women but shrink in response to pictures of nude men and infants. Women's pupils have the opposite response. Middle Eastern shopkeepers are said to observe the size of their customers' pupils when viewing precious jewels, enlargement indicating intense interest.

Most people favor one eye over the other, just as they favor one hand over the other. The one used most often can determine who strikes out in baseball. "Cross-dominant" batters who use right eye and left hand, or vice versa, can hit significantly better than those who use the same eye and hand. Pitchers, however, give up many more runs if they have the cross-dominant trait. The very best players are those who use both eyes equally, but this type of balanced vision occurs in only a small percentage of the population.

Muscles also protect the internal organs. The chest cavity is surrounded by bones, but the abdomen is not because the stomach enlarges after eating and a woman's uterus swells with pregnancy. Instead, the abdomen is protected by three layers of strong muscle.

Smooth muscles in the digestive tract contract, squeezing food and pushing it forward. Although the upper third of the esophagus is voluntary muscle that allows us to assist the beginning of the journey our food takes through 25 to 30 feet of intestine, the middle third is mixed and the lower third, just before the stomach, is entirely smooth muscle (Figure 2-2).

In the respiratory system, smooth muscles arranged in a circular pattern control the width of the air passages. Difficulty in breathing occurs if contraction is too severe, as during an asthma attack. Smooth muscle in the walls of blood vessels regulates blood pressure through the autonomic (self-controlling) nervous system. In the urinary tract, smooth muscle keeps urine flowing through the ureters from the kidneys to the bladder. Smooth muscle in the bladder wall contracts to expel urine. Where the urethra meets the bladder, a ringlike sphincter keeps the opening closed except during urination. A similar ring of skeletal muscle helps you control urination.

In a woman's reproductive system, smooth muscles in the fallopian tubes transport the egg cell from the ovary to the uterus. The uterus has very strong smooth muscle. By contracting, its muscles expel the uterine lining during menstruation and push the baby out during childbirth.

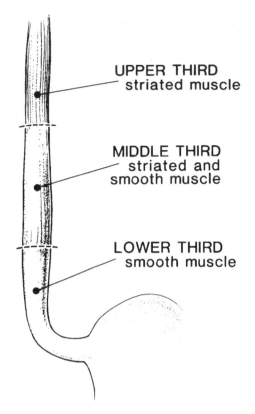

UPPER THIRD
striated muscle

MIDDLE THIRD
striated and
smooth muscle

LOWER THIRD
smooth muscle

FIGURE 2-2   Esophageal anatomy.

MUSCLE MISCELLANIA

The most variable muscle is the *platysma,* which lies in front of the neck. In some people, the whole area in the front of the neck is covered. In others, the muscle is straplike, and in a few people it is entirely missing. In the male gorilla, the platysma stretches to the groin so when he raises his arms in anger, his penis elevates and stiffens in sexual defiance. The longest group of muscles is the *erector spinae;* the widest is the external oblique muscle of the abdomen.

It is important to understand that all muscles are arranged to act as *levers.* The body uses three types of leverage systems—primary, secondary, and tertiary—depending on where the fulcrum (hinge or support) is located in relation to the force applied and the load moved (Figure 2-3). For example, in raising the

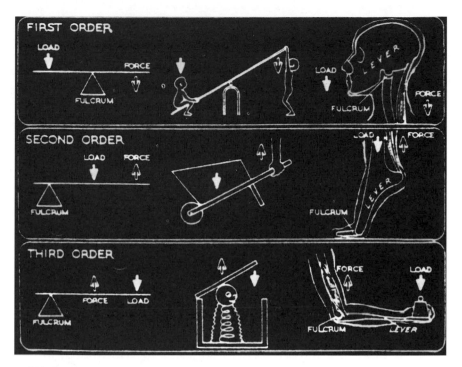

FIGURE 2-3   Lever systems.

forearm, the biceps pulls on the bone near the elbow. The fulcrum of this lever system is the elbow joint. The biceps applies a force and the forearm (the load) is elevated. The region between the fulcrum and the muscle, the *power area,* is almost always shorter than the load arm of the lever system. Because the lever magnifies the movement, the muscle only contracts by a fraction of an inch even though the forearm moves several inches.

More than 50 small muscles crisscross the face and head just under the skin. These produce a variety of facial expressions. Even though their movements are slight, they play an important role in producing facial expressions, of which there are seven universally recognized types: (1) neutral, (2) fear, (3) sadness, (4) happiness, (5) anger, (6) surprise, and (7) disgust.

The muscles that adjust the larynx to control speaking are tuned so that the pitch of the voice will rise sharply if the vocal cords are stretched by as little as 1 to 2 mm. Many of the body's muscles are arrayed about the hands and feet. Although they are very small and lack great strength, they can produce movements that are more delicate than larger muscles because they are served by additional nerves (the average nerve serves about 150 muscle fibers) to provide increased precision of control. For example, each eyeball has six muscles that work to tolerances of hundredths of an inch. They ensure accurate movements of the eye, and, the brain is kept informed about matters of distance and depth perception through their stretch sensors. Through the contraction of these six muscles, alone or in concert, the eye can be swiveled from side to side with great exactitude, moved up and down, and twisted clockwise and counterclockwise, or moved in any combination of these movements.

Muscles can be *anomalous,* or slightly unusual in their anatomy, in several ways. They can be duplicated. They can be absent. They can be split. The same is true of bones—one of every 20 people has an extra rib. This condition is most commonly found in men, and, according to the Smithsonian Institute, 7 percent of Japanese men and 16 percent of Eskimo men have an extra rib.

But enough of these generalities; let's take a closer look at how our bodies accomplish the amazing feat of movement.

3

The Structure of Muscle

"Anatomy is to physiology as geography to history:
It describes the theatre of events."

Jean Fernel (1497–1558)
On the Natural Part of Medicine

Muscle is a *contractile* system. As such, it requires a mechanism for contraction, a means of stimulating and regulating that mechanism, a source of energy to initiate and maintain contraction, a way of coupling this energy to the muscle, and a method for joining muscle to the bone to be moved.

The *ratio* of muscle to bone mass remains relatively constant (15 percent to 20 percent) throughout the arms and legs, even though the legs contain three times as much muscle and bone as the arms. The cross-sectional area of an individual muscle is inversely related to the length of its muscle fibers and directly related to its weight. The total cross-section of all the muscles in the human body is about six square feet. The maximal tension that a muscle can generate is equal to a force of approximately 45 pounds per square inch. If the one-quarter billion skeletal muscle fibers of the body all contracted maximally at the same time, they would produce a force of 25 tons.

CELLS

The cells (fibers) that make up all skeletal muscles are similar in structure. These fibers can shorten to approximately 60 percent of their resting length. Both the length of the muscle and the distance of its insertion from the joint it is to move control the degree to which a muscle can bend a joint (Figure 3-1). Athletic performance is often related to the lever arm length acted on by muscle. Because this and the overall length of muscle are fixed anatomic characteristics, this is an area in which heredity may affect skill, some individuals having dimensions more effective than others for the accomplishment of tasks such as lifting or throwing. Strength is also affected by the positioning of the muscles when contracting. For example, the biceps can lift a third more with the palms up (supinated) than with the palms down (pronated). This matter of greater contraction can make a profound difference in athletic performance. In 1957 Soviet high jumper Yuri Stepanov set a world record of seven feet one inch by wearing a shoe on his takeoff foot that lowered his heel, stretching his calf muscle and thereby giving him greater thrust on takeoff. Officials later prohibited its use.

Any pediatrician will tell you that adolescents tend to "outgrow their strength." During a growth spurt, the bones grow while the muscles lag behind, upsetting the ideal length–tension balance required for efficient movement. It was Galileo who over 300 years ago laid down the principle of similitude, or the scale effect. (Figure 3-2) He pointed out that for every unit linear increase in a

FIGURE 3-1 When b is greater than 25 percent of muscle length, full flexion is not possible.

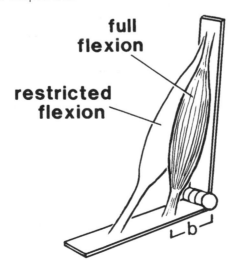

full flexion

restricted flexion

b

solid body (like an arm or leg), the surface area of the body increases by the square of the unit, its volume by the unit cubed. Ergo, a little growth produces a lot of mass that existing muscle may find difficult to move. Hence the "awkward" adolescent.

Nomenclature

Muscles are sometimes named because of their attachments (sternomastoid—running from the sternum at the front of the chest to the mastoid process behind the ear); action (radial flexors and extensors that bend or straighten the wrist); location (gluteus, the major muscle in the buttocks); structure (triceps, the three-headed muscle behind the upper arm); size (adductor magnus, the large muscle bringing the hip to the midline); or shape (deltoid, the shoulder muscle shaped like a Greek delta). A muscle occasionally bears an eponym, such as the muscle of Albinus (Bernhard Albinus, Professor of Anatomy at the Uni-

FIGURE 3-2   The scale effect.

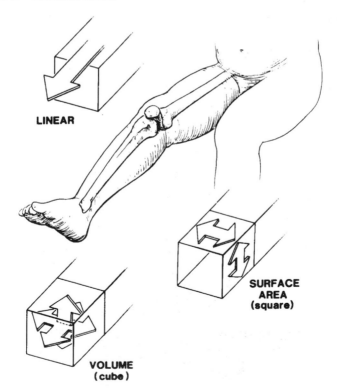

LINEAR

SURFACE
AREA
(square)

VOLUME
(cube)

versity of Leyden)—the rhomboid (diamond-shaped) muscle at the side of the nose, which he described in 1747.

The muscle bearing the longest name is the levator labii superioris alaeque nasi. This facial muscle connects your nostril and upper lip, and its contraction causes an "Elvis Presley" lip curl. The story goes that a professor of anatomy was invited by a colleague in another specialty to dine in the hall of an Oxford college. On arriving at table on this rather formal occasion, the anatomist was asked to say grace to the assembled fellows. Neither religious nor versed in the classics, he had no idea of any appropriate benediction. His wit, however, was as quick as his Latin was lacking, and, folding his hands reverently, he solemnly chanted: "Musculus levator labii superioris alaeque nasi." His fellow diners were suitably impressed by this novel supplication, and since then anatomists have known the muscle simply as the "grace muscle."

Fusiform (spindle-shaped) muscles (like the biceps—Popeye muscle—in the upper arm) have parallel fibers that are capable of quick spurts of activity over the greatest range of contraction. Penniform (feather-shaped) muscles, such as the deltoid muscle in the shoulder, provide multiple short fibers that can generate more tension per unit of whole muscle (Figure 3-3). Such muscles sacrifice speed for strength.

A single skeletal muscle cell is called a *muscle fiber.* The number of fibers in a muscle varies, depending mostly on its size;

FIGURE 3-3   Muscle shape can affect function.

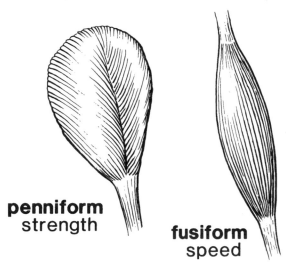

penniform
strength

fusiform
speed

for example, the biceps contain 2,600,000; the stapedius 1,500. Fibers are grouped into bundles called fascicles. Fiber thickness varies with the type of muscle. For example, ocular muscles have fine fibers, whereas the deltoid has coarse ones. Fiber diameter increases with age, exercise, and the influence of male sexual hormones. An adult fiber may grow to 10 times its diameter at birth, and exercise can further increase fiber size by up to 25 percent.

STRUCTURE

The muscle fiber in turn is composed of smaller elements called *myofibrils.* Each myofibril contains two types of filamentous subunits, one of which is thick and the other thin. These interdigitate in an overlapping array that produces a cross-striated banding effect as revealed by an electron microscope (Figure 3-4). They are arranged in a hexagonal lattice. The structural unit of a muscle fiber is the *sarcomere,* delimited by a "Z-line" at each end.

FIGURE 3-4   Muscle structure.

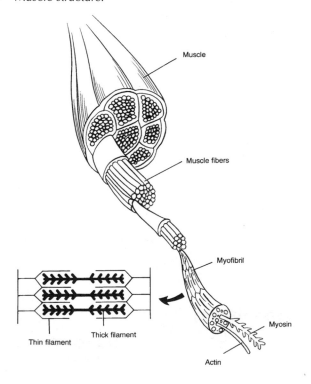

Microscopy reveals a repeating design of bands, zones, and lines within these sarcomeres, delineating overlap of the thick and thin filaments and producing the striped appearance of skeletal muscle. As we shall see when we look at the molecular basis for muscle contraction, the arrangement of these thick filaments and thin filaments is of prime importance.

All muscles are held together by thick fibrous tissue—the stuff you leave behind when you eat a good steak. This fibrous tissue gathers together at one end of a muscle, where it is fixed to a bone, and at the other end, where it forms a thick fibrous band called a tendon (sinew), which fastens to another bone. These attachments are called, respectively, the *origin* and *insertion* of the muscle. Tendons resemble ropes and, like ropes, the thicker they are, the greater the tensile strength of muscle and tendon. Tendons, by the way, are manufactured by *fibroblasts* ("fiber-makers"). These versatile, mobile cells extrude fiber molecules that self-assemble into long strands. The fiber that makes tendon so strong is triple-stranded collagen, twisted like a cable, white and glistening. When these collagen strands are arrayed in parallel, they provide maximum strength in the direction in which the muscle is pulling. Being fixed at both ends, shortening of the muscle will move any joint that lies between its origin and its insertion. Any muscle moving a joint is assisted by other muscles that stabilize the extremity and by antagonist muscles that work in an opposite function or as guy ropes to prevent violent and uncontrolled movements.

Tendons are slightly elastic to protect muscles and ligaments from excessive strain. The origin of a muscle—usually its stationary end—is firmly attached to bone by a short tendon. The insertion of a muscle—usually the end that moves—is attached by a longer tendon. For example, the muscles that move your toes are connected to your foot by long thin tendons that run across the front and back of your ankle. Bands of fibrous tissue (called *retinacula)* are wrapped around tendons at the wrist and ankle. They keep the tendons aligned so that they follow the correct direction of pull as they slide. Tendons are encased in sheaths *(synovial sheaths)* in places where they might rub against adjacent tissues. These contain the same membranes and lubricating fluid found in joints.

Just as the entire muscle is held in an envelope of fibrous tissue, so individual groups of muscle fibers are similarly contained. The fascial covering of the muscle itself is called the *epimysium*. Perimysium macroscopically subdivides muscle into fiber bundles (fasciculi), and endomysium surrounds individual muscle fibers (muscle cellular units) binding them together and to perimysium (Figure 3-5). Within this fibrous envelope the muscle cells are bathed in a fluid that contains the chemicals needed for contraction and relaxation. Access from the general circulatory system is through *microscopic tubules.* Blood vessels and nerves also enter this system.

Tiny spindles of highly specialized muscle cells served by nerves that regulate position are found throughout postural muscles. These muscle spindles register muscular tension so that fine postural adjustments can be made by the body where and when necessary. Another type of tension regulator is the *Golgi tendon organ receptor* found in tendons, which supplies

FIGURE 3-5   The fascial coverings of muscle.

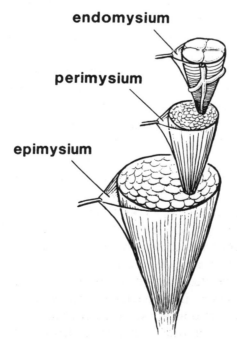

endomysium

perimysium

epimysium

the nervous system with information about muscle tension to prevent extremely forceful contractions that might separate tendon from bone.

In spite of variations in size and shape, all muscles have essentially the same structure. Myofibrils consist of muscle filaments arranged in a repeating pattern. Each unit of this pattern is called a sarcomere. Each sarcomere contains several types of filaments—thick ones containing the protein myosin, and thin ones containing the protein actin. About 100,000 myosin molecules laid side by side would form a ribbon 1 mm wide. Actin molecules are half as thick. The serial alignment of sarcomeres in adjacent myofibrils gives muscle fibers their striated (striped) appearance.

MOVEMENT

Although the movements initiated and controlled by muscle can be very complex, there are basically only three types of muscular action: (1) isometric, (2) concentric, and (3) eccentric. *Isometric* muscle action occurs when muscle exerts a force but neither shortens nor lengthens, as when you hold a heavy box in your arms. During *concentric* movement the muscle shortens. One example of this is lifting an object from a table, when the biceps muscle in the upper arm shortens to perform the lift. *Eccentric* muscle action occurs when the object is replaced on the table—the biceps lengthens as it creates force to avoid suddenly dropping the object. The various types of tension—concentric, isometric, and eccentric—all cooperate to provide balanced muscular action as we move through our day's activities. At the same time some muscles seem best suited to produce acceleration along the arc of motion of the joint (*spurt* muscles, such as the biceps in the upper arm). Others lie parallel to the long axis of moving bone and act to provide a stabilizing force during rapid movement (shunt muscles, such as the brachioradialis in the forearm) (Figure 3-6).

Muscles work together in pairs. The pull of one muscle can be counteracted by the pull of its opposite muscle. When a muscle contracts, its opposing muscle relaxes, which results in smooth movement (Figure 3-7). The natural tension of a muscle is muscle tone. Even at rest all muscles are in a partial state of

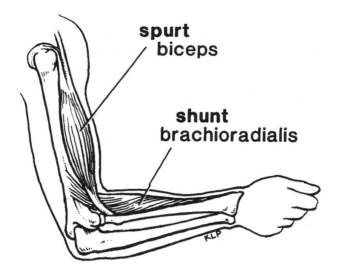

**spurt
biceps**

**shunt
brachioradialis**

FIGURE 3-6   Every muscle has a unique function.

contraction. This *resting tone* is necessary to control posture. When a person is lying down, his muscles are not relaxed completely. Only in a deeply unconscious state are the muscles entirely relaxed. Muscular rigidity with increased resistance to movement, called *spasticity,* can occur as the result of abnormally high muscle tone in disorders such as multiple sclerosis and cerebral palsy. On the other hand, *flaccidity,* or abnormally low muscle tone, is seen in disorders of muscle such as myasthenia gravis or muscular dystrophy (see Chapter 9).

PERFORMANCE

The engineering of the body allows it to accomplish some amazing feats. A good baseball pitcher can throw a baseball at over 90 mph, and gymnasts who form human pyramids can shoulder weights of more than 400 pounds. Great flexibility is possible in the joints of the limbs, and such suppleness can be increased with training. Yoga practitioners can wrap their feet behind their necks, ballet dancers leap and do splits, and acrobats perform incredible acts of balance. The great violinist-composer Nicolo Paganini (1782–1840) was reputed to have Ehlers-Danlos syndrome, a congenital condition of connective

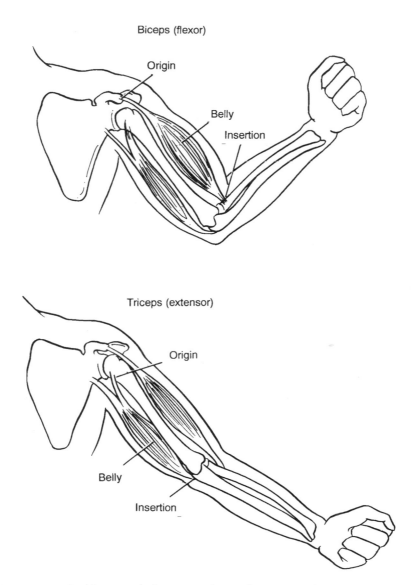

FIGURE 3-7   The biceps and triceps muscles work as antagonists.

tissue that results in hyperextensible joints and may have con-
tributed to his virtuosity as a performer. Paganini moved his
hand as flexibly as if it were without bones, which enabled him
to easily span three octaves on the violin.

Smokers sometimes claim that smoking relieves tension.
This may not be entirely psychological because nicotine can

reduce tendon reflexes. Folklore has it that during the Napoleonic era, lay medical practitioners in the mountainous regions of France would insert a cigar into a patient's rectum to obtain muscle relaxation and a measure of anesthesia. Certain foods can also influence our level of relaxation. Can it be an accident that "stressed" spelled backwards is "desserts"? Eating carbohydrate helps produce the amino acid *tryptophan*, which triggers the production of *serotonin*, a neurotransmitter that reduces pain and induces calm. Protein helps produce both dopamine and norepinephrine, which enhance alertness and concentration. Fat has no effect on serotonin, but it slows production of *dopamine* and *norepinephrine*. You can have the best of both worlds by eating chocolate, which has both sugar (carbohydrate) and fat. Besides, chocolate contains phenolethylamide, a substance associated with the release of endorphins (the body's natural painkillers) and is often linked with romantic feelings, as well as a dollop of theobromine, a stimulant similar to caffeine. Because of its taste and pharmacology, chocolate has a reputation as an aphrodisiac (from Aphrodite, the goddess of love). Montezuma, sixteenth century Aztec emperor and famed chocoholic, reportedly drank 50 cups of chocolate a day while visiting his harem of 600 women.

Involuntary muscle, such as that which controls our stomach and intestines, functions without any consciousness on our part. This is true of all the muscle found in our internal organs and cardiovascular systems. There is little we can do to significantly affect these muscles, which are under the control of our *autonomic nervous system*. However, biofeedback, meditation, and relaxation techniques can influence our internal environment to some extent.

Involuntary musculature is different in structure from its voluntary cousin. In the first place, it is not made up of fibers, but consists of spindle-shaped cells that are unstriated, or not striped. Each cell has a central nucleus and varies in length from 1/500 to 1/100 of an inch. Their width is even smaller (1/6000 to 1/4000 of an inch). These muscles can take on almost any shape, depending on their use. Although striated muscles are arranged in sections, the end walls of which provide anchoring points for the contractile forces produced by the gliding of their filaments, movement in smooth muscle results from a sliding action between their protein molecules.

Heart muscle is built like voluntary muscle but acts like the involuntary type. Whereas the nuclei in voluntary (skeletal/striated) muscle are arrayed underneath its membrane, those of cardiac muscle are centrally placed.

STRENGTH

Our strength is elusive. Examples of miraculous expression of power are well documented. We all have heard of the child trapped under the rear of the family car when the jack slipped during a tire change. His mother, tapping a source of strength far greater than any she would use in a normal situation, grabs the rear bumper and lifts the 3.5 thousand pound automobile off her son, who suffers nothing worse than a scratch or two.

At the same time muscle is remarkably adaptable. A fraction of an ounce of force is necessary for the muscles of the hand to pick up a pin or paper clip, about 5 to 6 pounds to hold a heavy book, and 30 pounds or so to lift a light suitcase. These same muscles can squeeze, with the dominant hand exerting more than 150 pounds of force. Well-delivered boxing punches land with the power of half a ton. The karate expert can break tissue and bone by imparting a large amount of momentum to a small area of his opponent's body. A well-executed karate strike that delivers several kilowatts of force over a few milliseconds will even break blocks of wood or concrete.

FORM

Muscle appears as a jellylike substance when it is completely relaxed. When called upon to contract, a drastic transformation takes place. In a few hundredths of a second, muscle changes into a hard elastic material with dynamic characteristics.

Muscle has a chemical basis similar to that of other body tissues. It is composed of approximately 80 percent water, 1 percent carbohydrate, 20 percent protein, and some fat and salt. Most other body tissues contain the same constituents in approximately the same ratio. Its special capacities result from the organization of its parts rather than from the materials that contribute to its construction. This organization enables a person to broad jump a distance of about twice his height. Special adaptations allow a kangaroo to bound about five times its height and the tiny flea to leap over a distance 200 times the length of its body (Figure 3-8). Where in the scheme of development did muscle originate, and how does it grow to move with such vigor?

FIGURE 3-8   Remarkable arrangements of muscle enable the kangaroo to jump five times its height and the tic to leap 200 times its length, while a man can only jump twice his height.

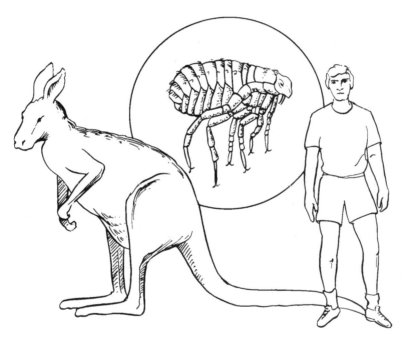

4

The Growth and Development of Muscle

"An organ is a cell state in which every cell is a citizen."

Rudolph Virchow (1821–1902)

Muscle develops from a group of cells called *mesenchyme* (middle layer). The outer membranes of these cells fuse at contact points during embryologic development, forming a single unit enclosed in a continuous membrane called a *myoblast* (*myo* = muscle, *blast* = formative cell). This early organization results in a so-called *myotube,* which in turn develops into an immature muscle cell that may contain hundreds of nuclei, one from each of the original cells. Further growth produces a mature muscle cell, or fiber, a long cylinder that measures 1/500 of an inch in diameter and several inches in length (Figure 4-1). Disruption of development at any point along this path can lead to a congenital disease of muscle.

FIBER TYPES

There are several distinct types of muscle cells, with a few sub-types as well. Cells generally are considered white (fast twitch) or red (slow twitch), as are muscles that contain somewhat more of one type or the other. A thin band of red muscle can be seen running along the sides of most fish. This alone is used when the fish is cruising. As any icthyophile knows, the bulk of the fish consists of pale muscle fibers, required only when speed is increased. The red color comes from the pigment *myoglobin,*

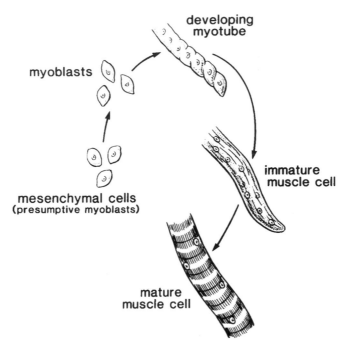

FIGURE 4-1   Skeletal muscle fiber development.

which provides the muscle with a store of oxygen for energy should its blood supply be shut off by its own contraction. This has to be replenished after a few seconds.

Muscles serving different functions contain different fiber types. *Postural* muscles such as the soleus (shaped like a flatfish) muscle in the calf that are programmed for continuous low level activity have a predominance of so-called slow-twitch fibers. In contrast, the muscles of the eye have a high percentage of fast-twitch fibers. The same holds true for animals. A greyhound is said to have only 3 percent to 5 percent of red fibers, whereas a mongrel may have up to 40 percent. The extraocular muscles are fast-twitch fibers because the eyes must move quickly for an animal to survive. On the other hand, the postural muscles of the legs that sustain the body in an upright position contain mostly slow-twitch fibers, which better sustain the upright body against gravity.

The motor nerve that serves the fiber determines whether it is a fast-twitch fiber or a slow-twitch fiber (Figure 4-2). To a certain extent, changes in function through exercise can alter

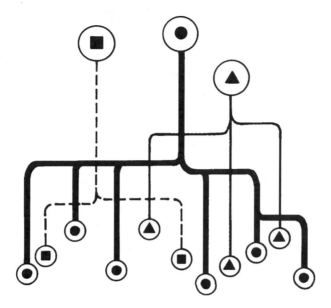

FIGURE 4-2   Three motor units and territories of innervation.

fiber type characteristics. The energy chemistry of the several types of muscle fibers is different in order to enhance the quality of either rapid or sustained contraction.

African Americans have a clear edge over Asians and Caucasians in athletic feats such as jumping or running. Coordination develops early in Blacks, as it does in Aborigines. Over 50 percent of NCAA basketball players are Black, although African Americans comprise only 11 percent of the U.S. population. Some Blacks have significantly longer arms and legs than Whites. Top Black Olympic sprinters have more fast-twitch fibers than Whites do. The muscles of Olympic champions such as Florence Griffith Joyner and Carl Lewis have more than 70 percent fast-twitch fibers. In contrast, Olympic marathon champion Joan Benoit Samuelson had 79 percent of the slow-twitch muscle fibers necessary for the endurance required in running a long slow race.

SKILLS

On the whole, animals outclass people in athletic ability. A man can run for brief periods at approximately 27 mph on a level surface and can run a mile at a speed of 15–16 mph. Almost every mammal of his size or larger can run faster, including hippos and rhinoceri, even on rough terrain. World-class jumpers can jump 7 feet in height or 29 feet or so in the long jump, but kangaroos jump higher than 7 feet, and impalas can beat the Olympic record for the long jump.

This is because we have only two legs, neither of which exerts much thrust most of the time. A quadripedal system is faster. We substituted two of our legs with arms that allow us to do wonders; however, no gymnast has ever matched a monkey as he swings through the rain forest canopy. Despite this, we are adept at many skills. We can not only run and jump, but also climb and swim. It has been said that a man can outwalk a horse. In 1882 George Littlewood walked 531 miles in six days. Compared with penguins, seals, and sharks, we are not very good swimmers, with a top speed of only 3.8 knots. Nonetheless, the English Channel has been swum both ways.

Although there are pentathlons and decathlons, most Olympic events are highly specialized and require a particular skill, ergo a specific physique. Shot-putters or javelin, discus, or hammer throwers require height and long arms. High jumpers must be tall. Gymnasts, as a rule, are short, which gives them a lower center of gravity and better balance. Some of these advantages are obviously mechanical—an object will travel farther if thrown from a greater height, and the longer the arm, the more momentum imparted at the moment of release. Except for the 100-meter dash (a special case), the longer the race, the shorter and lighter the runner. Athletes who require their arms to win are in a different category from those whose legs have to carry their bodies during a race. As a general rule, the longer the race, the older the competitors. The youngest athletes seem to be among the swimmers.

OXYGEN

Although record-breaking can almost be counted on at any Olympic games, sprint records are harder to beat than those of longer races. This is because increased training does little to improve "oxygen debt." All of the oxygen required for a 100-yard sprint is replaced *after* the race. Some athletes don't even bother to breathe during their brief dash, whereas others gasp only once.

In contrast, the runner in a mile-long race has to breathe 50 percent of the oxygen needed during the four minutes or so of the race, and training can improve this ability. It is only since the 1970s that it became possible to record running times in hundredths of a second. Unless we can improve on this technique, we may well be very close to the ultimate short-distance sprinting speed.

AFRICAN AMERICANS AND OTHER BLACKS

African Americans are noted for their excellence on the basketball court, but they also perform three times better in the Olympics than their population proportion would predict. The African Watusi has an average male height of almost 6.5 feet, with some of them as tall as 7 feet, and what seems to be a genetic passion for jumping. Jumps of over 7 feet under less than ideal circumstances are not uncommon. Because they lack other means of mobility, members of the Masai tribe are phenomenal walkers. Negro, in its strictest sense, refers to central, western, and southern Africans. Northern and eastern African dark-skinned people are considered as Hamites. Great Black distance runners such as Kipchoge Keino and Henry Rono are Hamites. Racial advantages would seem to give Negroes an edge in sprints and Hamites the advantage in long-distance running. The general order of "athletic efficiency" has been ranked as (1) African, (2) Asian, and (3) Caucasian.

Olympic records have fallen for several reasons. A larger group of world athletes is available for competition. Longer training periods and better training methods have also improved athletic ability. Many athletes competing in both the summer and the winter Olympics began hard training early in childhood.

WOMEN

Women are lighter and by and large have a weaker build than their male counterparts. On average, women's bodies have a smaller percentage weight of muscle and more fat, their legs are less muscular and shorter, their bones are smaller and lighter, and their total strength is less than that of men. Women's shoulders are narrower, their are hips wider, and they have a lower center of gravity. They also have a lower basal metabolism, with a male:female ratio of 141:100. They have smaller lungs and a smaller heart in proportion to the size of their bodies. Nonetheless, women have come to excel in all events in which they have participated, including basketball and ice hockey, which recently were added to the Olympic roster.

NERVE CONTROL

Although each fiber contracts in an "all-or-none" type of response to nerve stimulation, rarely are all muscle fibers activated at one time. Only the necessary nerve impulses to meet the need of the force required to accomplish a given task are sent, just a few to pick up a pencil, many more to lift a barbell. This is accomplished by a complex nervous feedback system based on the fact that muscular action will increase with increased load, just as a tractor engine is programmed to automatically speed up when the plow hits heavier ground. Such servo (feedback) control is required to keep us from expending as much energy lifting a fork as we would hoisting a 100-pound sack of concrete.

REPRODUCTION

Muscle cells pay for their specialized contractile ability. One of the things they cannot do is divide in order to reproduce themselves in the conventional manner of most cells. In humans and most other mammals, the number of muscle cells you have at birth is the number you have to work with as you grow. Muscle mass is increased through growth and exercise, by increasing the size of the existing cells. However, specialized *satellite cells* can regenerate muscle cells that have been damaged (Figure 4-3) through an intricate process of assembling structures already floating in the cell fluid. This is like rebuilding an old car from the scavenged parts of a number of wrecks. The muscle cell undergoes *necrosis* (death) and the satellite cell directs regeneration, which includes splitting of the nucleus and reduplication of the membrane containing the cell (the basal lamina). Eventually, however, the normal attrition that results from aging catches up with this

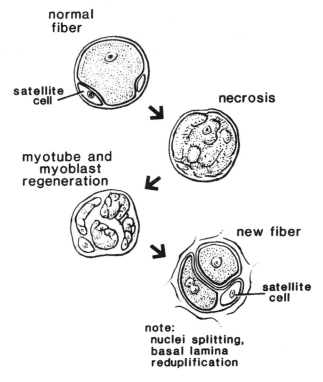

FIGURE 4-3   Satellite cell function with fiber splitting.

process. The weight of some muscles may decrease by as much as 30 percent between the ages of 35 and 75.

A number of things can accelerate loss of muscle. Stimulation to its muscle is cut off when a nerve is destroyed, as with polio, Lou Gehrig's disease (amyotrophic lateral sclerosis, or ALS), or trauma, and the muscle fiber becomes inactive, shrinks, and eventually is replaced by fat and connective tissue. The reverse situation results in a highly active muscle that increases in size and power. In this sense, muscular development can be looked upon as a direct product of muscle use.

ORGANIZATION

A single skeletal muscle can be thought of as a kind of living tension cable. It is packed with many hundreds of thousands of muscle fibers that form a pattern that is repeated down to the molecular level. Each of the fibers consists of 1,000 to 2,000 smaller strands called *fibrils* that run parallel to one another and are the contracting elements, the parts that do the actual work. These fibrils are about 1/25,000ths of an inch in diameter, and the space between them is filled with a fluid (cytoplasm). Densely packed within each fibril are hundreds of *filaments*, the smallest component of the muscle. When the cross-section of a fibril is magnified about 250,000 times under an electron microscope, these superfine filaments can be seen arranged in a geometric pattern in which the thin filaments and thick filaments alternate. Various lines, bands, and zones have been noted in the pattern and labeled (Z, I, A, M, H) for identification during microscopic examination (Figure 4-4). As the muscle fibril con-

FIGURE 4-4   Electron microscopic structure of muscle.

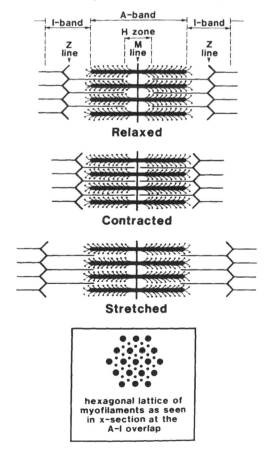

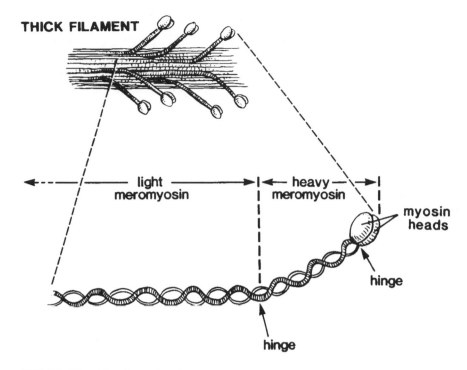

FIGURE 4-5   Myosin molecule.

tracts, the thin filaments slide between the thick filaments. Molecular arms on the thick (myosin) filament engage specific sites on the thin (actin) filament and by a sort of ratchet action shorten the fiber in contraction (Figure 4-5).

Now let's see how this mechanical process is electrically activated and chemically sustained.

5

How Muscle Functions

"Nature is sufficient in all for all."

Hippocrates (460?–377? B.C.)
Nutriment, XV (translation by W. H. S. Jones)

Much like an automobile engine, muscle utilizes both chemical and electrical forces to generate energy. The contraction (twitch) of a muscle fiber begins where its associated motor nerve is joined to its outer membrane, the *neuromuscular junction.* The motor nerve and the 50 to 400 muscle fibers it supplies is called the *motor unit.* The area where the motor nerve interfaces with the muscle cell is called the *motor end plate.* The bulbous end of the nerve at this point contains small sacs *(vesicles)* that contain a substance called acetylcholine (ACh), a "chemical mediator" that is released on arrival of the nerve impulse to induce contraction. At the point where the nerve contacts muscle, the membrane, including its lining (the *plasmalemma*), is folded into troughs *(synaptic folds)* that contain acetylcholine receptor sites. This is called the *end plate* (Figure 5-1). The nerve delivers a signal, called an *action potential,* whose transmission involves two sequences of electrical activity sandwiching an intervening chemical event.

NERVE STIMULATION

The process begins with a series of electrical pulses passed from the brain along various nerve fiber tracts in the spinal cord to the *peripheral nerve* that ends at the *neuromuscular*

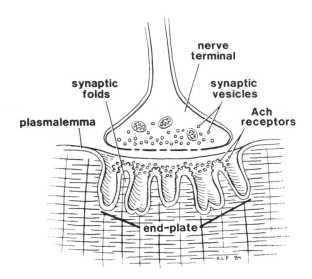

FIGURE 5-1   Neuromuscular junction.

junction (Figure 5-2). When the electrical pulses reach this junction, a chemical reaction is initiated that releases a squirt of acetylcholine. At the moment when the acetylcholine reaches its receptors on the muscle, the fiber is akin to a charged battery carrying an electrical charge of 0.09 volt. This is called the *resting potential* of muscle. Acetylcholine is a *neurohumor* (nervous system chemical secretion) that can temporarily change the molecular structure of the muscle membrane so that there is a two-way flow of potassium and sodium *ions* (an ion is an atom that is electrically charged) between the muscle cell and the fluid surrounding it. As these ions are exchanged through the membrane, the electrical balance of the muscle fiber changes (depolarizes) as it becomes temporarily discharged. This generates an *action potential,* an electrical discharge that spreads over the surface of the cell, transmitting a message through a tubular pathway called the T-tubules (Figure 5-3) to a holding area (the *terminal cistern*) within the membrane (*sarcoplasmic reticulum,* or SR) that surrounds the innermost contracting elements, the *myofibrils* (Figure 5-4). Finally, an interchange of calcium ions deep within the fibrils initiates contraction (Figure 5-5). The total time involved in a single muscle cell twitch,

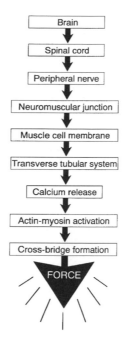

| Brain |
| Spinal cord |
| Peripheral nerve |
| Neuromuscular junction |
| Muscle cell membrane |
| Transverse tubular system |
| Calcium release |
| Actin-myosin activation |
| Cross-bridge formation |
| FORCE |

FIGURE 5-2   The nervous system is the communication network for the body.

FIGURE 5-3   T-tubule system.

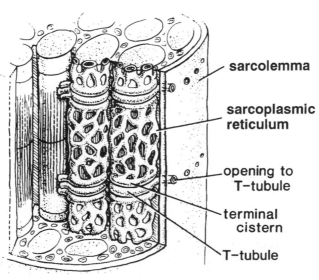

sarcolemma

sarcoplasmic reticulum

opening to T-tubule

terminal cistern

T-tubule

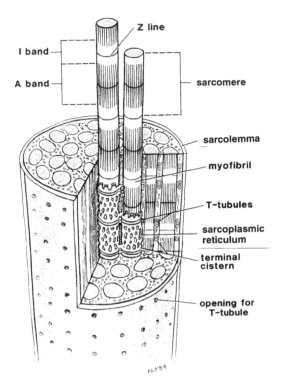

FIGURE 5-4   Relationship of T-tubule to muscle fiber.

including stimulation, contraction, and relaxation, is approximately 0.1 second.

Millions of muscle fibers are activated with every body movement. Electrical interactions with subsequent chemical changes constantly occur as electricity flows back and forth through the cell membranes and along pathways within the fibers. The "pacemakers" that orchestrate this activity are the nerve signals that release acetylcholine at multitudinal neuromuscular junctions.

Any disturbance at these junctions can have far-reaching effects. The lethal toxin of botulism as well as strychnine and cocaine all act by blocking chemical activity at the neuromuscular junction. These poisons can prove fatal by arresting the action of the muscles of respiration. However, in a weakened and refined state, miniscule amounts of botulinum toxin can block the action of specific muscles and relieve spasticity. Curare, another neuromuscular toxin, has been employed for

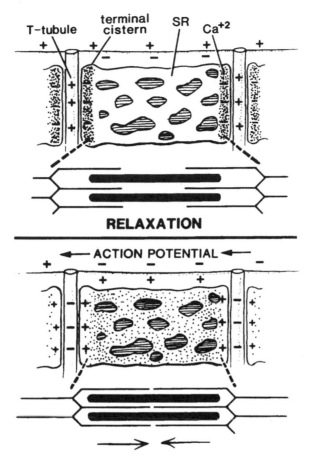

FIGURE 5-5   Muscle contraction initiated by nerve action potential with depolarization of muscle membrane.

years by peoples such as the African pygmies, to coat arrow tips or the darts used in blowguns to paralyze prey for easy capture. Succinylcholine, a potent muscle relaxant used in anesthesia, is a chemical cousin of curare. *Myasthenia gravis* is a disease in which patients suffer from muscular weakness and abnormal fatigue due to an abnormality in acetylcholine metabolism at the neuromuscular juncture. This disease counts Aristotle Onassis and Coach Weeb Eubank as two of its many victims (see Chapter 9).

With so much work to do, your muscles need a constant source of ready energy. What provides this?

6

The Energy
for Movement

"The cell never acts. It reacts."

Ernest Haekel (1834–1919)

Your internal-combustion automobile engine is driven by electrical sparks generated by its spark plugs. Muscle is moved by chemical "sparks" generated by the neurohumor acetylcholine (Ach) at the neuromuscular junction. The fuel for the automobile engine is gasoline. The fuel for muscle is adenosine triphosphate (ATP), the universal energy source for all living cells, plant as well as animal. Like all animal cells, muscle cells continually manufacture ATP from glucose.

As the term *triphosphate* indicates, the ATP molecule contains three phosphate (phosphorus plus oxygen) groups. They are hitched in line to the adenosine portion of the molecule. The energy in ATP is tied up in the force that bonds the last of these three phosphate groups to its brothers. This locked-up energy is released when, in the presence of water, the bond breaks, converting ATP to ADP (adenosine diphosphate) (Figure 6-1), and the third phosphate group is set free. The ATP molecule is like a tightly coiled spring, ready to release its energy when triggered.

MITOCHONDRIA

The powerhouses of the muscle cell are called *mitochondria*. They produce ATP through a complex sequence of chemical

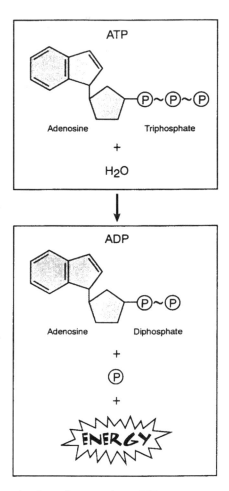

FIGURE 6-1   The production of energy from ATP.

events called the *Krebs cycle,* in which a variety of degradations and exchanges accompanied by the flow of electrons takes place to synthesize ATP.

Mitochondria are thought to have once been independent organisms that were captured by other cells for a symbiotic relationship in which they produce energy for the cell, in exchange for room and board. Incidentally, mitochondria have their own separate and unique DNA, called maternal DNA because it originated from the first human female and is passed on exclusively through the maternal genetic lineage.

Muscle has very high energy requirements and therefore contains many more mitochondria than are found in most other cells, and certain diseases of muscle occur because of defective mitochondrial metabolism.

AEROBIC AND ANAEROBIC METABOLISM

At rest only the *aerobic* pathway (the pathway that requires oxygen) is in operation. *Anaerobic glycolysis* (which does not use oxygen) is the primary energy source for vigorous activity lasting from 30 to 90 seconds. It produces less ATP than the aerobic process but produces it much faster. For sustained exercise, *oxidative phosphorylation* is the method of choice because it slowly produces considerably more ATP than the anaerobic process.

Lactic acid is an end-product of anaerobic metabolism during periods of vigorous exercise. This is because during periods of extreme exertion a process very much like fermentation takes place inside muscle cells. Nature, being very efficient, recycles this lactic acid to produce more ATP. The capacity of the anaerobic system to produce energy without oxygen is, of necessity, limited, and the body's oxygen balance must be settled sooner or later. That is why an athlete breathes very deeply after a strenuous run. He is paying off the "oxygen debt" that his muscle cells incurred during anaerobic metabolism.

The Krebs cycle requires oxygen for its function. During vigorous activity the body's oxygen demands sometimes exceed its supply. A highly trained athlete can respire enough to supply his blood with 7 to 8 pints of oxygen each minute. The heart must pump more than 20 quarts of blood each minute to distribute this oxygen throughout the body. This is about the most that the cardiorespiratory system can provide. When this limit is reached, the Krebs cycle cannot keep up with demand because of lack of oxygen and the cell must produce ATP in an anaerobic (*an* = without, *aerobic* = oxygen) fashion. The Krebs cycle is bypassed and ATP is produced by a chemical process called *glycolysis*. The Krebs cycle begins to operate normally when oxygen again becomes available.

EXCITATION CONTRACTION

When the muscle cell is at rest, all the elements for contraction are there and available, including ATP, but no contraction occurs because calcium ions remain isolated in a special compartment of the cell where they are kept away from muscle fibrils. As soon as the electrical action signal spreads over the cell membrane, calcium is released and the actin and myosin filaments begin to slide. Cycles of contraction and relaxation depend on the alternate loosening and re-forming of the bonds linking actin to myosin so that the filaments are pulled past one another. This is governed by two clever molecules, *troponin* and *tropomyosin* (Figure 6-2), which work together to expose

FIGURE 6-2   Troponin and tropomyosin located on the actin molecule.

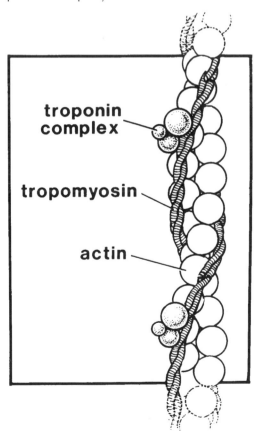

troponin
complex

tropomyosin

actin

myosin-actin binding sites during contraction and to block them during relaxation (Figure 6-3).

The bonds in an active muscle must be loosened and re-formed from 50 to 100 times a second for smooth contraction to occur. As you can see, the central nervous system (brain and spinal cord) works very closely with muscle. If you simply *imagine* that you are lifting a heavy weight or scaling a wall, tensions will be generated in appropriate muscles even though there is no actual movement. Your eyes move during "rapid eye movement" under closed eyelids when you are dreaming, and they tend to move up and down when the dreams involve rising or falling objects, and from side to side when something moves across your inner field of vision.

CENTRAL NERVOUS SYSTEM CONTROL

If muscular movement were not controlled by the central nervous system, certain muscles would bend your arms and legs,

FIGURE 6-3   Troponin and tropomyosin at work exposing myosin-actin binding sites during contraction.

RELAXATION

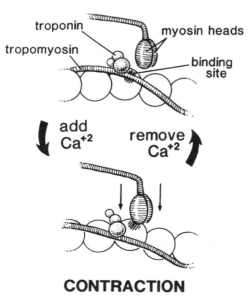

CONTRACTION

while others would tend to straighten your limbs and hold them stiff as ramrods (Figure 6-4). To prevent this, the muscles are arrayed in the body in pairs with opposing action. These are held in equilibrium and automatically monitored by the *cerebellum*,

FIGURE 6-4   From brain to muscle—the sequence of movement.

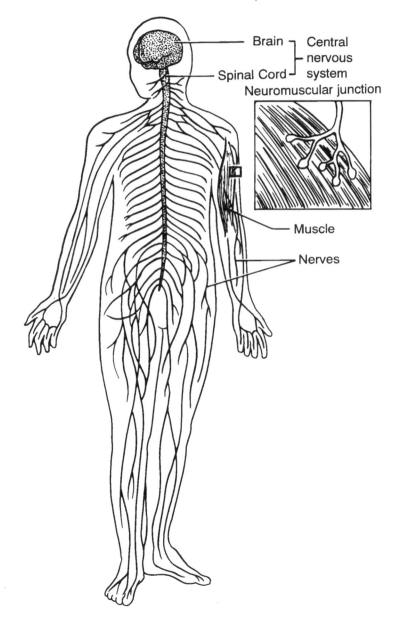

the brain center at the back of the brain that is concerned with stability and balance. Gently rocking a baby stimulates its cerebellum. The more rocking, the earlier the baby develops coordinated movements and the faster he or she will grow and mature.

Our brains determine and monitor other important motor abilities, such as handedness. The lowest forms of life showing brain dominance are birds, which have neuronal populations in their left hemisphere that regulate their song production. The question is why are some of us left-handed? Studies have indicated that babies who usually lie with their head to the right become right-handed; those who turn to the left become left-handed. This is one of many theories to explain dominance, none of which make much sense. However, most cases of left-handedness are thought to be caused by minor brain damage due to reduced oxygen supply before or during birth. There is no scientific evidence to support this opinion, only statistics. For example, twins, who have a high proportion of neurologic problems due to crowding in utero, are almost twice as likely to be left-handed as single births. People with epilepsy, people who are mentally retarded, and children with learning disorders are disproportionately left-handed. Autistics have the highest population of left-handedness; 63% favor their left hand over their right. Many conditions, such as allergy, migraines, stuttering, dyslexia, thyroid problems, and skeletal deformities, are experienced more by those who are left-handed.

On the other hand (no pun intended), the incidence of left-handedness is also higher than average among the world's great artists, including Michelangelo and Leonardo da Vinci. Benjamin Franklin was a southpaw, as were one of four astronauts (as compared to the incidence of 1 of 10 in the general population), and the list goes on. One distinct advantage of left-handedness is that almost 40 percent of lefties use both sides of the brain to process speech instead of the left side only, as right-handed people do, so they recover speech loss from strokes better than righties.

REPAIR

Regeneration of damaged muscle may be complete or may fail, leaving the surrounding basement membrane empty. Defective fusion of regenerative cells leads to a *myopathic* (muscle disease–like) configuration. Imperfect healing may leave a narrowed or *atrophic* segment in the muscle (Figure 6-5). Scientists are currently investigating the repair and regeneration of muscle cells in the hope that such studies may indicate a way of making damaged muscles heal faster, or even replacing dead muscle with fresh muscle transplanted from another source. Such techniques could be particularly useful in open heart surgery. Research in this area depends increasingly on the work of biologists concerned with the basic science of muscle function.

Investigators are studying chemical compounds that simulate the behavior of muscle fibers. Their ultimate goal is the conversion of chemical energy to mechanical energy without intermediate steps.

FIGURE 6-5   Muscle fiber regeneration.

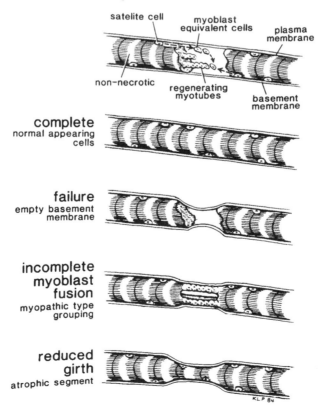

The evolution of cellular movement consists of a continual refinement of the inherent properties of the simplest cells. What we learn about muscle cells provides insight into the structure of all living matter.

Now that we have some idea how muscle works, we'll take a look at this marvelous tissue in action. Let's discuss exercise.

7

The Exercise Prescription

"The wise for cure on exercise depend . . ."

Epistle to John Dryden of Chesterton (1700), Line 92

All children have an inborn imperative to move. Even though it is well established that motor nerves are not fully developed until the age of 4 or 5 years and sometimes even later, physical stimulation through exercise can help a child develop motor skills such as coordination much earlier. Patterns of movement can be stimulated and motor activity facilitated in newborns and infants to assist them in developing self-awareness through movement. Muscle strengthening will help a child master the ability to sit. Making the infant aware of the role and support of his feet assists him or her in standing, and walking is encouraged by balancing exercise. One such program is the system of graduated exercise that begins with relaxation and then incorporates gymnastics in preparation for sitting and movement to prepare for standing as well as exercise play in preparation for independent movement, as developed by Dr. Janine Lévy *(The Baby Exercise Book,* Pantheon Books, 1973).

AGING

It has been said that if exercise were available in a pill, it would be prescribed for almost every patient and every medical condition. Muscular activity is necessary for protein synthesis, and simply keeping up with the normal muscular loss due to aging (called sarcopenia) requires the exercise prescription. It is well known that, with complete bed rest, strength is lost at approximately 3 percent each day. The total number of muscle fibers declines after age 30, reducing muscle strength by up to 30 percent at age 60. Between the ages of 30 and 80 the strength of the leg, arm, and back muscles can decrease as much as 60 percent, reflecting a progressive decrement of muscle, with as much as 10 percent to 15 percent loss per decade after age 50.

Neuromuscular changes and decreased levels of body hormones are in part responsible for this deterioration, but the major contributor is reduced exercise, particularly heavy loaded exercise. Endurance also suffers, which leads to fatigue. Studies in animals have found that the ability of muscles to provide sustained power diminishes with age by 50 percent. This appears to be due to a loss of mitochondria, which in turn results in a decline in enzyme-linked oxidative capacity. Older muscles are more easily injured and take longer to recover. Protracted healing lengthens the period of immobility due to pain. Muscles rapidly lose strength with complete bed rest and normal power may never return. Such weakened muscles are vulnerable to injury, thus initiating a vicious cycle of weakness–injury–pain–weakness.

Aerobic capacity also decreases with age, resulting in a reduction of muscular vigor. This physiologic decline begins at about age 30. From then on the ability of the heart to pump declines by approximately 1 percent a year. Blood vessels are nearly 30 percent narrower by middle age, decreasing blood flow in the limbs by 30 percent to 60 percent by age 60. After age 30, the force of gravity overpowers weakening muscles in the stomach and back, leading to a gradual compression of the intervertebral discs that results in a decrease in height. In addition, the tensile strength of ligaments is diminished, which adds to injury propensity in the elderly.

BENEFITS

The good news is that this trend can be reversed through exercise! Numerous studies have shown that graded, well-supervised exercise programs, including both aerobic and strength training, can lead to significant functional improvement in such parameters as gait velocity, stair climbing, and spontaneous physical activity in middle-agers and even in individuals over 70 years of age. Regular exercise reduces premature mortality from cardiovascular disease and has been proven significantly protective against *ischemic* (reduced blood supply) strokes. Lifelong regular exercise may also guard against the development of Alzheimer's disease.

Exercise also helps keep the body trim. Fat is our primary fuel, and one pound of fat provides 3,500 calories. It is difficult to burn that off at "one fell swoop" unless you run a marathon, because the muscles use sugar before they tap into fat for energy. Actually our bodies are extremely efficient in converting food into fuel. For example, riding a bicycle at 10 mph for one hour requires only three ounces of carbohydrate. This is the energy equivalent of about 1.4 ounces of gasoline. If we used gasoline instead of food, we could ride more than 900 miles on a single gallon! Sugar is stored in the muscles, utilized more easily, and therefore recruited first. But there is not very much sugar immediately available, so it runs out quickly. In contrast, fat is stored at a distance from the muscles and is harder to access when you first start to exercise, but fat is absolutely inexhaustible. Ultimately, both sugar and fat provide the energy used to make ATP, and the energy from ATP is then used to contract muscles.

ENERGY SYSTEMS

Muscles run on ATP, and there are three ways to make it. The first is through the aerobic system, which is oxygen-dependent and provides endless energy. This system burns sugar and fat and makes large quantities of ATP, but provides it only slowly. Therefore, aerobic metabolism is used for sustained exercise such as a long, slow jog.

The second method is what is called the *lactate system*. It makes less ATP but provides it very quickly. It is an anaerobic (no oxygen necessary) arrangement that is called upon to provide energy for a brief but intense effort, such as a 5 to 7 minute sprint. The lactate system burns only sugar and that is why it runs out of energy quickly.

The third way to produce ATP is through the creatine-phosphate (phosphagen) system. This lasts only a matter of seconds and provides only small amounts of ATP, but it provides it very quickly. The ATP comes from stored ADP (adenosine diphosphate) and creatine phosphate inside the muscle. This process does not require oxygen, fat, or sugar to function.

Thus the creatine-P system is used for intense but brief activities such as the 100-yard dash. For events longer than the 100-yard dash but shorter than a mile, the lactate system produces energy, and for activities that last longer than approximately seven minutes, oxygen is the critical factor (thus the term *aerobic*). Such exercise can last for many hours with the slow oxidation of fat and sugar. As described in the last chapter, the lactate system produces lactic acid as an end product. This causes the burning sensation in the limbs that occurs with intense exercise and remains until the lactate is remetabolized.

LOSING FAT

Exercise helps you lose fat because it increases the body's use of calories. One hour of vigorous activity can burn up to 600 calories—the equivalent of a milkshake and a hamburger. A 150-pound individual will burn up 13.2 calories by vigorously running for one minute, 8.1 calories by swimming, and 6.35 calories by bicycling. Aerobic exercise utilizes 6.6 calories per minute, whereas walking uses only 3.8 calories in the same time. A 150-pound person chopping with an ax at a fast pace for one hour will burn up 1,212 calories, cross-country skiing 486, golfing 348, performing judo 798, playing basketball 564, and playing billiards 174 calories.

Exercise builds lean body mass as it burns excess fatty tissue. It keeps the percentage of body fat at an appropriate level. Exercise can decrease appetite, although it usually increases thirst. It may help to remember that the feeling of being hungry sometimes be satiated by drinking, particularly a warm fluid such as weak tea. Finally, exercise increases the body's rate of metabolism for up to six hours, so that you continue to expend more calories after as well as during your exercise period.

A German proverb claims "He who goes for a walk lengthens the way to his grave." Exercise indeed improves every organ in the body.

❏ The liver responds by producing glycogen more efficiently.
❏ Insulin and glucose are better regulated by the pancreas.
❏ More oxygen is delivered by the lungs and the heart pumps stronger.
❏ The circulatory system builds more capillaries.
❏ The level of "bad" cholesterol (low-density lipoprotein, or LDL) in the blood drops, while the level of "good" cholesterol (high density lipoprotein, or HDL) increases.
❏ Bones respond by becoming denser.
❏ The mitochondria that produce ATP enlarge and increase.
❏ The muscles learn to burn more and more fat.

Here are some myths about exercise that should be dispelled.

1. *If a little exercise is good, more must be better.* People over 60 need exercise to only 70 percent of their capacity to derive maximum benefits. Overexercising is not practical and may be dangerous.
2. *Exercise leaves you fatigued and in pain.* An unsupervised binge of exercising can, of course, exhaust you and make your muscles sore. Well-scheduled regular exercise relaxes you and increases energy.
3. *Exercise can cause a heart attack.* A sudden burst of intense exercise after years of sedentary living *may* put strain on your heart. However, reasonable regular exercise develops a healthier heart and can ward off a heart attack.
4. *Hard work can make you age.* Working so hard that you can barely drag yourself to bed will wear anyone out, but a regular exercise program produces changes in the body that slow the aging process.
5. *For exercise to be effective, you have to work out many hours each day.* Studies have shown that exercise two to

three times a week for a minimum of 20 to 30 minutes is all that is necessary to maintain fitness.

There are three components to a complete exercise program. You will require

❑ *Endurance* exercises that are aerobic in nature. These will condition your cardiovascular system and lungs and help you relax. They may include a walking or jogging regimen.
❑ *Strengthening* exercises are necessary for posture and balance. Selected calisthenics are recommended.
❑ *Range of motion* exercises, including stretching, will improve joint mobility.

SCHEDULING

The best time to exercise is usually in the morning or late afternoon. Midday may be a poor choice in the summer because of the warm weather. Aerobic capacity, muscle strength, and flexibility are all at their peak between 3 P.M. and 4 P.M. A minimum of three and a maximum of five workouts each week is adequate. Workouts can be performed anywhere. The bedroom is a good site for stretching exercises. Carpeting may provide enough padding, or you may want to purchase an exercise mat. Walking and jogging should be done in the most pleasant surroundings possible. Proper running shoes must be worn, and it is best to run on springy turf or cinder if at all possible. You can exercise year-round if you wear appropriate clothing. You undoubtedly will find your workout particularly invigorating in moderately cold weather. Apparel should be loose and layered for outdoor exercise so that the outer layer can be peeled off as you warm up and sweat. You must sweat if you are to benefit from exercising.

It is important to check with your doctor before beginning any exercise program. If you make any significant changes in your level of physical activity, you should check with your doctor again. Remember to take it slow in the beginning and determine your limit. This means exercising at a rate that is within your capacity. You should warm up before you work out in order to increase blood flow to your muscles. This gradual startup helps prevent injury because soft tissues are most easily damaged when they are cold. You should cool down after the workout because your circulatory system needs to readjust. Usually three to five minutes of walking after a jog will suffice. Do not shower immediately after exercising. A hot shower can open up the circulation just as vigorous activity does. Delay your post-workout shower at least 5 to 10 minutes and, even then, make the shower warm, not excessively hot. If you exercise with others, do not compete and never overexert yourself. Overdoing stimulates adrenaline, which decreases the efficiency of the heart. Finally, do not exercise if you are sick because exercise challenges your body to reach its full potential. If you have even a slight cold, your physiology has enough to do without overloading it with exercise. Eat lightly before exercising, but do not skip meals because your body requires nutrition to fuel its activity.

BODY TYPES

Somatotyping identifies physique by considering shape, not size. It was developed by William Sheldon in 1940 by looking at the body types of 4,000 American college students. There are three basic body types—endomorph, mesomorph, and ectomorph. Endomorphs are rounded, like pears. Mesomorphs look like models, with broad shoulders, narrow hips, and a lot of muscle. Ectomorphs are tall and thin (Figure 7-1). Everyone has a little bit of all three body types but with one dominating. An exercise program can shape you up, but it is impossible to change your basic body type. Although the average population varies widely in body type, certain somatotypes are better for certain sports. Endomorphs are essentially out of the running; mesomorphs or ectomorphs, or combinations thereof, are in preponderance. In other words, it's not just "drive" and practice that wins events. It's mostly what shape you are in (no pun intended). For example, shot-put competitors are mostly mesomorphic, whereas runners are less powerful, thinner, and tend toward ectomorphic stature.

An athlete's "high" and so-called "second wind" are due to neuropeptides such as encephalins and endorphins, secreted by the brain, which act as tranquilizers after about 10 minutes of continuous exercise. Highly trained athletes "run through" the

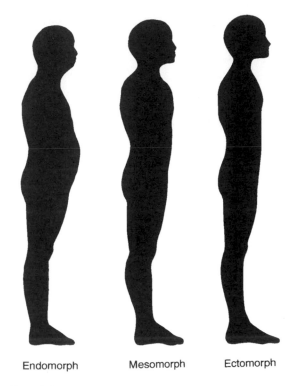

Endomorph   Mesomorph   Ectomorph

FIGURE 7-1   Somatotypes.

brief walls of pain and fatigue they encounter—you and I should stop when we experience severe fatigue or our exercise hurts.

SOME EXERCISE POINTERS

- ❏ Do not bounce during stretching.
- ❏ Avoid vigorous overarching of the back and do not exercise with your knees locked.
- ❏ All muscles act in sets, and exercise should be aimed at balancing the use of these muscle pairs.
- ❏ Stretching and strengthening muscles is the object of proper exercise.
- ❏ Pay attention while you are exercising. Develop muscle awareness. Let your body guide you.
- ❏ Remember that movement is natural and has a healing quality. Nowadays patients are encouraged to move within 24 hours after surgery.

❏ During stretching, stretch just a bit beyond the point of fatigue.
❏ Do not exercise too fast or you will overload your joints.
❏ Avoid deep knee bends or stretch situps or pushups.

TAKING THE EXERCISE PRESCRIPTION

It is never too early and rarely too late to begin an exercise program to prevent or even reverse age-related problems. Exercise is effective in maintaining proper joint nutrition and mobility in degenerative arthritis. Aerobic exercise is beneficial in reducing the risk of cardiopulmonary illness and improving general fitness. A long-term goal of 30 minutes of brisk walking or other aerobic exercise at least three times a week is ideal. Regular walking with a partner keeps you both motivated. If you can hold a normal conversation without getting out of breath while you are walking, your pace is just about right. If walking is too strenuous, you can exercise from a chair to start. Moving rhythmically while seated provides aerobic exercise. Chair "dancing" is a gentle but active alternative exercise program. (For information contact Chair Dancing, Dept. P, 2658 Del Mar Heights Road, Del Mar, CA 92014; phone 800-551-4386.)

It is not necessary to carry hand weights while walking—they don't increase muscle strength and although they add a bit of aerobic intensity to the walk, walking faster or walking uphill has the same effect on the heart. If you insist on using hand weights, make sure that they do not weigh more than three pounds. The use of heavier weights stresses your neck, shoulders, and arms. Avoid ankle weights because they can alter your gait, making you injury-prone. Both strength training and a program to enhance flexibility contribute to increasing and maintaining function.

Resistance exercise should be initiated with very light loads. Lifting exercises should be done rapidly because they will increase your ability to perform the explosive movements that are necessary to rise from a chair or catch your balance. It is reasonable to allow six weeks before changes become noticeable. If you expect immediate dramatic improvement, you will become discouraged and discontinue your exercise regimen.

A complete program of strengthening can be designed with a modest investment in very simple equipment, such as plastic-coated dumbbells, elastic bands, and ankle weights. A stationary exercise bicycle, stepmaster, or cross-country ski machine will provide adequate resistance and endurance training. A treadmill can substitute for a vigorous walk in inclement weather. Walking in waist-high water in a swimming pool will provide effective resistance, and water aerobics are an excellent form of exercise, particularly for senior citizens.

Balance Exercises

Balance exercises as simple as alternately standing on each foot or the use of a wobble board stimulate proprioceptive feedback (tactile and position sense) through *mechanoreceptors* arrayed about joints. For this reason, exercising on a moving bicycle is better than the same amount of peddling on a stationary bike, because the ability to balance is necessary for the activity. Research studies have shown that nursing home residents who enrolled in a program of balancing exercises including Tai Chi (slow Oriental drill) movements suffered far fewer falls with subsequent broken bones than those who did not participate.

We lose "functional reserve" as we grow older, and every year approximately 30 percent of people over age 65 and 50 percent of those over 80 fall. Almost 10 percent of those who fall are seriously hurt. Other risk factors include poor vision and loss of feeling in the feet. In addition to balancing exercises, here are some other things you can do to reduce your risk of falling.

❑ Make certain you have good lighting in your home.
❑ Wear low-heeled shoes with soles that provide good traction (see chart for more details)
❑ Clean your floors of clutter, loose throw rugs, and electric cords.
❑ Have your doctor check for postural hypotension, a condition in which blood pressure drops when you stand up.
❑ Make sure you are not taking any drugs that could make you drowsy, dizzy, or light-headed.
❑ Be especially careful in winter. Avoid icy or slippery sidewalks and stairs.

The balance reflex mechanism can always be improved. Therapies and preventive measures are available to anyone with balance problems. Balance exercise can be as simple as standing at a sink holding on at the sides, rising on tiptoes, and then slowly lowering yourself. You can practice getting out of a chair four to five times without using your hands or making it a goal to walk a little further each day. The American Physical Therapy Association is a good resource for information to help seniors avoid falls and get answers to questions about their balance. (American Physical Therapy Association, 1111 N. Fairfax St., Alexandria, Virginia 22314; 703/684-2982; Fax 703-684-7343.)

SENIOR SHOE SAFETY

1. Purchase new shoes at the end of the day because your feet may swell after the day's activities.

2. Wear only properly fitted shoes. Avoid high-style shoes that do not conform to the natural shape of your foot. Wearing shoes that are uncomfortable increases your risk of an accident.

3. Do not expect to "break in" a new pair of shoes. They should be comfortable when you first try them on.

4. The heel of the shoe should not slip. This could cause a heel blister.

5. Avoid heavily cushioned shoes. They can cause instability.

6. Do not wear shoes with smooth rubber or leather soles when walking on wet or slippery surfaces.

7. Heavily worn heels and soles provide unstable support. Replace them in a timely fashion.

8. Shoes should provide good traction yet be light and fit snugly.

9. Soles with heavy lugs can catch on carpeting and cause a fall. They should be avoided.

10. Shoes with tied laces can be adjusted to accommodate bony protuberances or swelling. They do not tend to fall off the foot and are safer than shoes without laces.

11. High-heeled shoes not only cause bunions and hammertoes, but also significantly increase knee strain, which may cause degenerative changes in the joint, leading to osteoarthritis. Perhaps this is one reason osteoarthritis of the knee is twice as common in women as in men. The moral of the story is "women, wear flats!"

Stretching

Limbering up by stretching is a necessary component of any exercise program. Stretching maintains flexibility, which helps to avoid injury and enhances daily function. Flexibility can help you avoid surgery or other medical treatment. A podiatric study of more than 100 people who complained of foot pain concluded that many who were advised to have surgical corrective procedures could avoid such operations if they regularly stretched their Achilles tendons. Much low back pain can be prevented or eliminated by properly stretching the muscles of the low back and the hamstring muscles on the back of the thighs (Figure 7-2).

FIGURE 7-2 Exercises for the back.

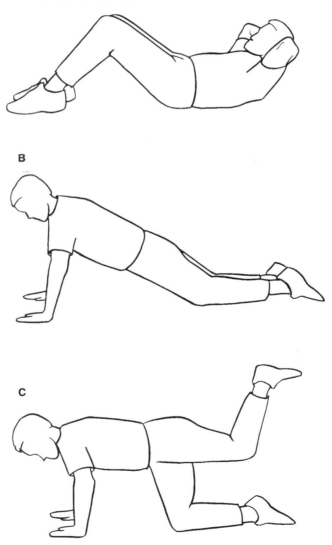

STRETCHING EXERCISES FOR THE BACK

A. Abdominal Curl—Lie on your back with feet flat on the floor and knees bent. Interlock fingers and put hands behind your head. Tuck your chin and lift your shoulders off the floor. Tighten abdominal muscles and hold for a moment. Slowly bring shoulders back down. Relax a second and repeat. Work up to several sets of 10-15 repetitions each, resting for a minute or two between sets.

B. Modified Push Up—Lie face down on floor with palms flat and just to the sides of your shoulders with your elbows bent. With knees on the floor, slowly push your chest up. Stop when elbows are about to lock. Hold for a second, then return to the starting position. Work up to two sets of 10-15 repetitions, resting a minute or two between sets.

C. Cat stretch—Kneel on the floor with palms flat and arms stretched directly below the shoulders. The knees should be hip-width apart. Slowly lift one leg, knee still bent, so that you raise your thigh a bit higher than your trunk. The sole of your foot should be facing the ceiling. Hold for a moment. Breathe normally as you feel the contraction in your low back and buttocks. Slowly return to starting position. Repeat with other leg. Work up to two sets of 10-15 repetitions (one repetition entails lifting right and left leg), resting for a moment between each set.

When should you stretch? If possible, both before and after exercising. Although you might feel a gentle pull, stretching should not hurt. The admonition "no pain, no gain" should be buried. Do not bounce when you stretch, and by all means do not have someone else passively force the stretch beyond your pain threshold. Each stretch should be held for 30 seconds. Stretching beyond that brief period adds no benefit. You should, of course, slowly work up to the 30 seconds if you cannot reach that level the first time you stretch.

Osteoarthritis of the knee currently afflicts some three million Americans, mostly those over the age of 60. This condition responds to exercise. It has long been thought that people with osteoarthritis of the knee have weak quadriceps (upper leg) muscles as a result of the disease. The theory was that the pain caused by the arthritis prevented people from moving about and that the muscles wasted with disuse. It now appears that weak thigh muscles are a *cause* rather than a *result* of osteoarthritis of the knee. People with a strong quadriceps are able to control how hard they impact with the ground when they walk. In so doing, they reduce stress on the knees. Those with a weak quadriceps lack this control and tend to impact harder when they walk or run. Unnecessary stress is placed on the knee, leading to a breakdown of the cartilage that cushions the joint. Loss of joint alignment occurs, and proprioception (joint position sense) is decreased, initiating a vicious cycle of further damage. In carefully controlled studies a program of quadriceps strengthening exercise resulted in significant improvement in patients with osteoarthritis of the knee.

Exercise videos are helpful in initiating and following an exercise program. Many are currently available. I suggest that you borrow some from your local library and see which suits your particular time and need. The Jane Fonda video is very popular for aerobic exercise and the Karen Voight fitness videos, especially the ones on stretching, have garnered positive reviews from exercise scientists.

Two- to four-pound plastic-covered dumbbells are excellent for exercising the forearms and shoulders. A modified pushup (with the knees on the floor) can be quite effective in building strength in the shoulders. The legs have the largest muscles in the body, and they should be exercised for stamina and to help burn more calories. Squats are intended to strengthen the quadriceps muscles. When squatting, you should bend no further than 90 degrees. Deep knee bends are forbidden!

Believe it or not, sexual activity is an efficient calorie burner. A 125-pound woman can burn up to 4.5 calories per minute during intercourse. Sexual activity also enhances muscle tone and is a great cardiovascular workout. Heart rate can reach 125 beats per minute during sex.

An alert person can find many opportunities to exercise during his or her daily routine. Here are some suggestions. Take every opportunity to walk. Without even trying, the average person will walk 115,000 miles in his lifetime, or 4.5 times around the world! So you've got a good start. Now continue your round-the-world marathon by walking whenever you can. Walk up and down stairs instead of taking elevators. It has been estimated that each stair you climb adds four seconds to your life. Lift and carry reasonable loads rather than using wheelbarrows or carts (but always remember proper technique lifting—from the knees and not the back). Tighten your abdomen, attempt to bring your navel to your backbone, and hold it for a slow count of six when you are driving and have to wait for the stoplight to change. Perform simple isometric exercises at your desk each day. This involves contracting muscle without moving joints, in contrast to isotonic contraction in which joints are moved. This could include pressing your hands together, pulling your hands apart, pressing your knees together, pushing your knees apart against the resistance provided by your hands, lifting yourself by your hands in a firm chair, pushing away from your desk, bending your head to each side against resistance provided by an outstretched palm, and so forth. Each of these isometric positions should be held to a slow count of six. You will have to use 75 percent of your strength before you get any benefit, so try to exert a maximal contraction when exercising isometrically like this (Figure 7-3).

Aerobic Exercise

An anonymous wag once said, "I have two doctors—my left leg and my right." Indeed, aerobic exercise affects the entire body. It improves your lungs, liver, heart, and bones; increases endurance; and enhances general health. To be effective, aerobic exercise must use the muscles of the legs, make your heart beat faster, and induce deep breathing. Uninterrupted exercise for about 15 min-

FIGURE 7-3   Isotonic versus isometric contraction.

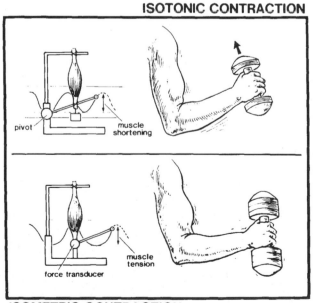

ISOTONIC CONTRACTION

ISOMETRIC CONTRACTION

utes is ideal, but you can gain aerobic benefits simply by running in place as fast as you can for one to three minutes. This works your legs, makes you breathe deeply, and increases your heart rate. You always continue to metabolize fat after exercise, but you only metabolize fat *while* exercising if the exercise is aerobic.

The heart is a highly specialized muscle. It contracts like any other muscle, metabolizes fat, and depends on glycogen for energy. The body has a mechanism that preferentially directs its metabolism to replenish glycogen for the heart before other muscles are served. Even though the blood may be loaded with glucose, other muscles do not get any until the needs of the heart are satisfied. Other muscles receive glycogen only after the heart's glycogen is replenished. If any sugar is left over, the glycogen storehouse in the liver begins to fill. No one knows how this mechanism works. It is another example of the mystery and the miracle of the human body.

Active Rest

Recovery after injury often is not hastened by rest because injured joints are particularly vulnerable to long absence from movement. Without exercise, soft tissue about a joint tightens, causing pain when motion is attempted. For this reason, a program of "active rest" has been proposed by sports medicine professionals. This seeks a balance between the activity that has caused the injury and underuse, which is likely to worsen it. Active rest for a running injury of the knee might be swimming or walking. Active rest for a strained back involves special exercises and returning to work (assuming that you are not a professional furniture mover). Varying your exercise program provides the brief periods of rest that muscles need.

Sphincter Exercise

Exercise is even effective in increasing the tone of some internal sphincter muscles—the circular muscles that guard the openings from our bowel and bladder. The doughnut-shaped muscle that tightens to prevent urine leaking from the bladder can be strengthened by an isometric exercise that involves squeezing the sphincter shut as if to hold in the urine and keeping it tight for three to five seconds. This can be repeated frequently during the day. It is also effective to perform the squeezes while urinating. After letting out some urine, you should stop the flow for a count of four and then continue urinating until your bladder is entirely empty.

Increasing Strength

Recent studies have shown that a two-month strengthening program in men and women aged 60 to 96 increased the strength of the 60-year-old and 70-year-olds by 200 percent and the size of their muscles by 15 percent. Those in their nineties experienced a 180 percent gain in strength, while their muscles grew by 12 percent. In addition, their bones became denser.

Weak muscles are poorly supplied with oxygen. They tire easily when you attempt to work them, and they ache and want to rest. Muscular exhaustion occurs because muscle fibers run out of the oxygen needed to extract energy from sugar and fat. Working a muscle builds circulation so that more oxygen is delivered to the muscle factory. Strength and endurance increase, and limbs that are stronger allow you to avoid accidents, from dropping things to stumbling and breaking bones.

A muscle's ability to use oxygen and fuel increases with an increase in temperature. That is why warming up before exercise is important. Additionally, because warm muscles are more elastic, they are less susceptible to injury. Higher temperatures also improve the function of nerves. As the capillaries in the muscles dilate with warming, more blood carrying more oxygen is brought to the muscles for the removal of waste products such as carbon dioxide and lactic acid. The heart also benefits from warming up. Cardiac irregularities on an electrocardiogram often are decreased by warming up. Finally, fat is burned more efficiently in muscles that have been warmed up.

Recent scientific studies have shown that strength training does not cause women to become muscle-bound. Instead, such training reduces body fat. A slight increase in weight may occur because lean body mass weighs more than fat. However, while strength training results in increased strength, there is no significant increase in lower body girth and only a slight increase in the size of the upper extremities. Women should be encouraged to train at high intensity because light training often is below what is necessary for physiologic adaptation in body tissues. Finally, women can use the same training methods as men because they are no more likely to be injured during strength training. Sport-specific exercise should take into consideration the biomechanics of the sport for which a woman athlete is training.

Some of the strength-training benefits for women include higher metabolic rate, increased functional strength for daily activity and athletic participation, decreased body fat, increased lean body muscle mass, stronger connective tissues (ligaments and tendons), increased bone modeling and strength with a subsequent reduction in the risk of osteoporosis, and enhanced confidence and self-esteem.

Natural Exercise

Natural exercise provides benefits that exercising on a machine does not. Besides being more fun, outdoor exercise calls upon the body to balance and adds a cross-training effect. If you run on a trail rather than on a treadmill, you have to adjust to irregularities in the running surface, and even sometimes run uphill, which gives a wind-sprint effect. It is best to walk or jog with occasional short bursts of effort in the middle. These spurts of intensity tend to burn fat more efficiently.

Cross-Training

Because the nerves that carry sensations from one limb to the spine connect with nerves that carry sensations down into the opposite limb, exercising one limb will improve muscular function in its mate. In fact, exercising the legs can even cause changes in the arms because exercising the lower limbs induces *systemic* effects (blood, liver, heart) that increase performance in the upper limbs. The opposite effect, exercising the arms, has little effect on the legs because the arm musculature is relatively small compared with that of the legs.

Muscle fibers enlarge in response to demand. A muscle will enlarge if it is contracted long enough, often enough, and hard enough. It will do this without hormones and without protein in the diet because it gets preferential access to amino acids and uses available protein in the body for muscle synthesis.

Eastern Exercises

Eastern exercise techniques have become very popular. *Tai Chi* is a very relaxing exercise that involves the performance of slow, formalized dancelike movements. It is a relaxation technique that includes a meditative quality. The best way to start a Tai Chi program is to find an instructor and join a group. You can check out a book from your local library to get some idea of what is involved. There also are excellent videotapes that are easy to follow.

Yoga exercises are a pleasant way of stretching, relaxing, and meditating, all at the same time. The various positions—called *asanas*—gently stretch and relax the body. Proper breathing techniques are important during these exercises. Source materials are books and videotapes. Although it is possible to teach yourself yoga, it usually is better to join a class at your local health club or community center to get started, and then carry on by yourself if you wish.

Tae Bo combines Eastern martial art techniques with aerobic exercises. It provides a rigorous workout. Videotapes are available for rental or purchase.

Special Techniques

Special exercising techniques such as the Alexander method, which emphasizes balance of body segments, or the Feldenkreis technique, which is directed toward balancing the right side against the left side of the body by correcting the imbalance caused by handedness, are available as physical therapy treatment when indicated for special postural problems. *Isokinetic exercise,* using special machines that progressively load a joint through its arc of movement, is often prescribed for special athletic training. More details on fitness, including illustrated instructions for specific exercises, can be found in my book, *All About Bone: An Owner's Manual* (New York: Demos Medical Publishing, Inc., 1998).

It has been said that exercise is to the body what reading is to the mind, and I hope by now I have convinced you of its benefits. An interesting bit of trivia is that you exercise 45 facial muscles by frowning and it takes only the risorius and zygomaticus in tandem with 15 other muscles in the face to smile. I am not suggesting that you stop smiling and frown instead just to exercise your face. By all means keep smiling. And a program of regular exercise should help you do just that.

8

Injury to Muscle, Ligaments, and Tendons

"What wound did ever heal but by degrees?"

William Shakespeare (1564–1616)
Othello, II, iii, 377

Musculoskeletal soft tissue injuries are more common than broken bones. Sprains, strains, and contusions account for almost 40,000 days lost from school or work and more than 500,000 hospital discharges. All such injuries are caused by stress, ranging from a simple single overload to chronic overuse.

MUSCLE TENSION

Muscle tension frequently results from anxiety, feeling "uptight," or other emotional stress. Each year more than $300 million is spent on tranquilizers and sedatives to soothe fraying American nerves. If you doubt this, just listen to how common language reflects our tendency to somatosize resentment or irritation. "You're a pain in the neck," we say, or "Get off my back." When a situation is too vexing, our response is, "I can't shoulder this." And how many times have you heard "This job is a humongous headache!"

Then again, stress is not always negative. The happiest moments in life—reunions, births, weddings, retirements—are enormously stressful. But our bodies cannot differentiate between negative and positive stress, between "stimulating" anxiety and genuine threat. Stress, as defined by Dr. Hans

Selye, who devoted his life to its study, is defined as "the non-specific response of the body to any demand made upon it." Whatever the demand, the body reacts with a "general adaption syndrome" alarm that includes a rapid pulse, dry mouth, sweaty palms, and tightening of the muscles, particularly those about the face and neck. Blood vessels constrict, the pulse begins to race, and blood pressure rises. Blood lactate increases, indicating widespread muscle contraction. Metabolism gradually returns to normal but if the stress is perpetuated, normal functioning cannot be maintained and only a small amount of additional stress can cause a "nervous breakdown."

This pattern of "fight or flight" served our Stone Age ancestors well. Modern living usually does not require either of these extreme reactions, and many of our greatest stresses, such as divorce, changing a job, relocating a home, or suffering the death of a spouse, relative, or close friend, require relaxation rather than physical mobilization. Exercise can be a part of this relaxation formula because it builds up energy, inhibits tension, and decreases fatigue. It does this by increasing glycogen, the fuel for physical activity in the muscles, by increasing oxygen available to the muscles for more intense activity, by conditioning muscles so that they can do more before becoming fatigued, and by slowing the rate at which fatigued muscles recruit others to accomplish a given task. Other relaxation techniques are outlined elsewhere in this book. These include Tai Chi, yoga, stretching, and meditation. Massage also is useful in relaxing muscles. Deep massage relieves muscle soreness by activating touch and sensation nerve fibers. The functioning of these fibers tends to "jam" the nerve impulses generated by smaller pain fibers so you do not feel as sore.

STRAIN AND SPRAIN

The terms *strain* and *sprain* are often used interchangeably. This is incorrect. A strain is an injury to a tendon or muscle, whereas a sprain refers to disruption of a ligament. Ligaments hold joints together. They are elastic but they stretch and tend to stay that way when stressed. Our ligamentous skeleton is built for mobility rather than stability. After stretching to 6 percent more than its resting length, a ligament builds up considerable passive tension and begins to tear (Figure 8-1). Sprains are classified according to severity. A grade I sprain is a stretched ligament, grade II is a partial tear, and grade III is a complete disruption.

Our *locomotive unit*—the pelvis and lower limbs—consists of 57 muscles and 11 joints, which means that we have a good

FIGURE 8-1   How a ligament heals.

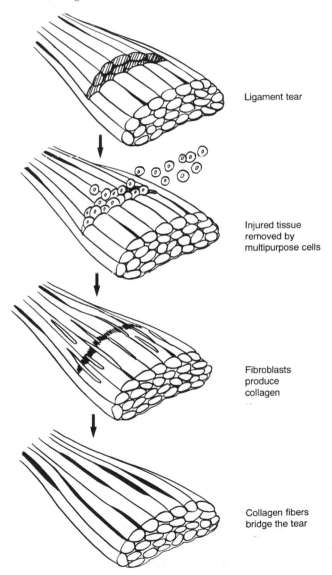

Ligament tear

Injured tissue
removed by
multipurpose cells

Fibroblasts
produce
collagen

Collagen fibers
bridge the tear

statistical possibility for injury. The ligaments of the ankle and knee joints are put under considerable stress during athletic activity and are therefore particularly prone to damage. The outside of the ankle is less stable than the inside of the joint and usually is sprained by twisting the foot inward on the leg. Rotation injuries of the leg with the foot firmly planted are a common cause of knee sprain.

Sprains usually are managed with a treatment program called R.I.C.E.—**R**est, **I**ce, **C**ompressive wrap, and **E**levation of the injured part. Some severe sprains require a plaster cast or brace to immobilize the involved joint. Complete rupture of a ligament may sometimes require surgical repair. This is particularly true for the ligaments that stabilize the knee, which include the anterior cruciate, the posterior cruciate, the posterior lateral ligament complex, and the medial and lateral collateral ligaments.

Muscle begins to weaken and atrophy almost immediately after injury. For example, the muscles that fully straighten the knee (those along the inside border of the thigh) can lose up to 25 percent of their strength within the first 48 hours after damage to this joint. It is enervating to walk in a crouched position, and it requires twice the force to fully straighten the knee as it does to bring it to within the last 15 degrees of extension. Rehabilitation of the joint through appropriate exercise is important from the onset of treatment.

MUSCLE DAMAGE

A *contusion* is a soft tissue injury that is caused by a direct blow to a muscle. Bleeding may occur if the damage is severe enough. This results in bruising of the skin and underlying soft tissues. Swelling ensues, and calcium deposition with deep muscle scarring and joint stiffness may occur in severe injuries.

Bony formation sometimes occurs following muscle damage. This is called *myositis ossificans* (muscle inflammation—bone formation). Such bone may restrict motion by decreasing elasticity in the involved muscle or by obstructing movement of a joint. The diagnosis of myositis ossificans is made by an appropriate history, physical examination, and imaging [x-ray, computed tomographic scan (CT), magnetic resonance imaging (MRI)] to reveal the bony deposit. R.I.C.E. after trauma can control bleeding, which decreases the incidence of bone formation. Physical therapy is not appropriate after bone has formed because it can cause additional trauma and the formation of still more unwanted bone. The bone can be excised (removed) if the condition is painful or disabling, but only after the bony mass has completely matured, which may take three to six months. Premature removal could result in a recurrence that might be even more extensive than the original condition.

Ectopic ossification (bone formation) can complicate injury or surgery, particularly in patients with a neurologic disease such as cerebral palsy or paraplegia secondary to spinal cord injury. In these cases the bone is laid down in the tissue planes between muscles—often around the hip, where it can cause locking of the joint. Preventive treatment includes nonsteroidal antiinflammatory drugs such as ibuprofen, diphosphenates (which inhibit bone formation), and radiotherapy.

Cardiac muscle and smooth muscle do not regenerate; they are repaired by scar formation. Skeletal muscle has greater reparative power, the extent of regeneration depending on the type of injury. In an incised wound with little loss of substance, muscle cells proliferate to form bands that bridge the gap and eventually become striated muscle. If muscle fiber has been destroyed, the damaged remains are removed by special cells called *macrophages*, and the gap is closed by fibrous tissue, which then matures into a scar. Tendon has very little blood supply so that healing occurs very slowly, but it may be remarkably complete. If the gap in a damaged tendon is small, it eventually can fill completely with tendon cells. However, if it is large, scar tissue must be used.

When voluntary muscle atrophies, its fibers shrink. If the disuse is permanent, its contractile elements may be converted to fatty and fibrous tissue. Degenerative changes due to inflammation, such as that seen in typhoid fever, the pneumonia of epidemic influenza, and following measles, may cause a specific degeneration described as a *hyaline change*. This involves a remarkable swelling of the cells, which eventually lose their striations and become amorphous, homogeneous, and granular. However, regeneration of this muscle may be remarkably complete, with the entire muscle renewed.

TENDON TRANSFER

Muscle can be transferred for reconstructive purposes as long as its blood supply remains intact. *Tendon transfer* is a not uncommon orthopaedic procedure that is used to substitute a functioning muscle for one that has been lost after an injury to nerve or muscle. This reconstructive procedure is used in people who have cerebral spastic palsy or have had poliomyelitis, or in any other condition in which it is necessary to substitute a good muscle for a bad one. Questions of function, length, and tension have to be addressed in selecting an appropriate tendon for transfer.

Techniques vary, but it is usual to select a muscle that has the same or similar strength and function as the one for which it will substitute. Muscles become "hard-wired" regarding their nerve supply and function. A muscle that pushes the foot down is not the best substitute for one that pulls the foot up.

Free tendons (detached at both ends) may be used for tendon grafts, as either an *autograft* (from the body of the patient) or an *allograft* (from another human body, usually a cadaver). Other allograft tissues include ligament, fascia, and, of course, bone. Proper storing (usually freezing or freeze-drying) as well as adverse immunologic response to foreign tissue are considerations in the use of an allograft.

Nonbiologic substitutes for ligaments and tendons are also available. These include carbon-impregnated woven synthetics as well as silk and other materials.

STIFFNESS

We seem to stiffen with age and complain of more pain in our muscles. The cause of this stiffness and soreness usually is not in the joints themselves but in the muscles, ligaments, and connective tissue that move with our joints. Our tendons and ligaments become less extensible with age. These structures shorten if they are not stretched to improve joint mobility, placing undue pressure on adjacent nerves. Pain is then transmitted by nerve impulses traveling along these pressured pathways.

PAIN

The body's reaction to a cramp is to automatically immobilize the muscle by making it contract. This response is called the *splinting reflex*. In this way, a sore muscle can set off a vicious cycle of pain, splinting, contracture, more pain, more splinting, and so on. This cycle of discomfort is common in painful conditions of the lower back. In addition, a muscle that is overworked becomes fatigued and cannot fully relax. Blood flow becomes restricted in areas of a muscle that are in spasm. Such relatively inadequate blood flow (ischemia) can itself cause pain. This distress triggers the splinting reflex and further contraction of the muscle, which induces the pain cycle. Relief requires a break in the cycle, usually provided by gentle but forceful static stretch to break the muscle spasm and relieve the pain.

Using a muscle in an abnormal position can initiate cramping and pain. Long hours of close work, never allowing the neck to fully extend, results in stretching of the muscles in the back of the neck with shortening of the muscles in the front. The improper use of bifocal or trifocal eyeglasses can cause neck strain with muscle spasm. Gentle stretching exercises are the best prevention and/or treatment for these problems because they lengthen muscles that have contracted as a result of pain and decrease the electrical activity in them, thereby relieving the discomfort caused by muscle spasm.

STRAINS

Muscle strains frequently involve biarticulate (two-jointed) muscular structures. These muscles work in an "eccentric" fashion, in which the muscle fibers produce force while lengthening, as in lowering a barbell or running downhill. The hamstring muscle group on the back of the thighs, so called as the tendons of these muscles are severed when an animal such as a bull is "hamstrung" in order to cripple it, most commonly is involved in athletes because these muscles move both the hip and the knee. The actual location of such injuries appears to be primarily at the muscle–tendon junction and presents as a local inflammation. The cardinal signs of inflammation are present—

calor (heat), rubor (redness), turgor (swelling), and dolor (pain). Chemicals such as *prostaglandins,* which stimulate pain nerve endings, gather at the site. Histamine is secreted to dilate blood capillaries in the vicinity, making them "leakier" than usual. Increased blood flow to the inflamed area causes the redness that you see and the heat that you feel. All of this accelerates cellular activity to expedite healing. Plasma leaks from the capillaries, causing swelling, and the inflammatory process attracts fibroblasts, which set to work repairing damaged tissue.

Strains can be minimized by warming up before exercise. Physiologic warming increases the length and elasticity of the muscle–tendon unit. If a muscle's strength and temperature are increased, protection from stretch (strain) is enhanced. Preconditioned muscles require more force to failure and stretch farther from their resting length before weakening, demonstrating a relative increase in elasticity and providing some measure of strain prevention. The muscle–tendon unit is essentially an energy-absorption system. Muscle that is contracted is capable of storing more energy before failure than is noncontracted muscle.

Muscle aching and soreness usually are overuse symptoms that improve with rehydration, massage, and rest. However, unusually intense or abnormally prolonged exercise may result in *rhabdomyolysis* (dissolution of muscle), which can overload the circulation with debris from damaged muscle (e.g., myoglobin), leading to kidney failure. Severe muscle soreness can reflect a generalized disorder of metabolism and/or produce laboratory findings that mimic a heart attack or even liver disease.

Muscle soreness is related to cellular changes that produce inflammation and edema (swelling), as noted previously. A severe muscle cramp is commonly called a "charley horse" (from horse racing slang, "we are indebted to the turf when an attack of rheumatism is denominated a 'dose of the Charley-horse.'"—H. Spencer, colloq.) and results from a sudden nerve discharge that contracts the entire muscle belly. Dehydration after prolonged exercise is a significant risk factor for muscle cramp. Heat, rest, and massage may help to relieve cramping.

Chronic cramping can lead to gradual shortening of the entire muscle, and, of course, the ultimate contracture is the sustained rigidity seen in rigor mortis after death. Although muscles can be electrically stimulated to contract for several hours after death, they begin to lose their tone by approximately

2 to 4 hours post mortem, progressing to complete rigidity in about 12 hours. This is because, lacking the energy to contract, the muscle fibers lock in place. By observing the degree of rigidity and the position of the body in rigor mortis, a coroner can estimate the time and place of death. After a few hours (in less time with heat) rigor slowly disappears as the muscle undergoes enzymatic autolysis (spontaneous disintegration) until the limbs again are flexible.

CRAMPS

Muscle cramps can disable even the fittest of athletes. In 1989 Michael Chang sustained painful thigh cramps during his heroic defeat of Ivan Lendl at the French Open tennis competition. The 17-year-old player drank water between points, massaged and stretched his legs, and ate bananas (to replenish potassium) during breaks. Chang's cramps decreased and he went on to score one of the more notable upsets in tennis history.

The terms *cramp* and *spasm* often are used interchangeably to refer to a sustained, painful, involuntary muscle contraction. Some people get cramps because of a low serum glucose level. They also can be caused by fluid loss or electrolyte imbalance, overexertion, or inadequate conditioning. Injury and fatigue can play a role. Although cramps may affect athletes who are in excellent condition, the poorly conditioned person who sporadically attempts a high level of exercise is at the greatest risk. A "stitch" refers to a sudden, sharp pain in the side or abdomen. This occurs during exercise (usually running) if you are out of condition. A stitch is caused when the body diverts blood to actively exercising muscles. This temporarily starves the abdominal muscles of blood, producing a spasm that causes a painful "stitch."

Both stretching and pressure are effective in treating cramps. Drinking water is the best treatment because fluid deficiency appears to be a primary cause. Salt tablets not only will not help, but also may actually be harmful because salt draws fluid out of the circulation and into the stomach. It can also irritate the stomach lining, leading to greater discomfort. Among the many touted treatments for cramps in athletes is pinching the upper lip. This pinch must be strong enough to almost cause discomfort. It probably works because it causes some alteration in neurotransmission to the muscle. Ice is the preferred treatment for most cases of acute muscle cramp because it causes the muscle to relax. Potassium-rich foods such as bananas and oranges are also helpful.

Cramps may have nothing to do with activity. Instead, they may simply be symptomatic of such medical problems as rheumatoid diseases, diabetes, arteriosclerosis, endocrine disorders, or any other condition that interferes with muscle metabolism or affects circulation. Prevention is the rule. In professional sports the emphasis is on proper hydration and adequate clothing. Elite cyclists always have a support team to supply plenty of drink, and you see baseball pitchers sitting in the dugout wearing warm-up jackets to keep their circulation going.

CREATINE KINASE

Serum creatine kinase (CK), the key enzyme in the muscle's energy system, leaks from the tissue during muscle damage, and its blood level may be dramatically elevated. Runners are particularly prone to elevated CK levels, which can rise to 10 to 15 times normal (2 to 200 depending on the method of testing) after a marathon. Cyclists, swimmers, rowers, and cross-country skiers have lower post-exercise CK levels. But at any time athletes can have serum enzyme levels two to three times those of sedentary people of the same age or sex. A form of CK is also present after cardiac muscle damage resulting from a heart attack. This confuses the diagnosis of a heart attack in an athlete with a high CK level from skeletal muscle damage. Other tests (electrocardiogram, radionuclide imaging) can clarify this situation. Prolonged strenuous exercise also may be associated with transient elevations of skeletal muscle enzymes that are also present in the liver. Hepatitis can be ruled out by other examinations of liver function.

DELAYED EXERCISE PAIN

Delayed exercise pain is the stiff, tender feeling that comes on several days after exercise and makes your muscles hurt for a day or so. This delayed muscle pain may be due to small tears in the muscle or to a change of the pH (acidity) of muscle fluids.

Injured muscle fibers become more permeable, allowing substances that should not to leak in and out. One of these is calcium, and an elevation of calcium within a muscle cell wreaks havoc on the chemistry of the cell.

The best way to stop delayed muscle pain is to do a gentler version of the exercise that initiated it. Adhesions from an injury may be stretched and broken, and endorphins (natural pain killers) serve to lessen these symptoms. The "gating" mechanism, by which the activity of one set of nerve fibers closes the gate and shuts out signals from another set of fibers, also operates in this situation. Smaller pain fibers are activated when muscle is damaged. Performing a gentler version of the same exercise to relieve delayed muscle pain produces friction and heat in sore muscles, which may trigger large nerve fibers to modulate the pain sensation of the smaller fibers. Rubbing the area increases touch sensation, which also activates larger nerve fibers, closing the gate and dampening the activity of the small pain fibers. Massage can be enhanced by the use of liniments and ointments for muscle soreness. This technique is called *counterirritation*.

PROCESSING PAIN

An example may help you understand this. Let's say you stub your big toe hard. Ouch! At first you feel a sharp pain. The A-delta nerve fibers that carry the electrical signal to the spinal cord at about 40 miles per hour have just kicked in (no pun intended). Then you begin to feel a throbbing ache that slowly spreads up your foot. This is due to activity of the C-fibers, which carry their message to the spinal cord at approximately 3 miles per hour. The difference in speed may account for perceived variation in the quality of pain. The final sensation of discomfort you experience is a blend of the separate nerve responses.

Next, touch and pressure sensations are sent to the spinal cord by A-beta fibers at some 180 to 200 miles per hour. These messages race to the spinal cord where they block the incoming stimulation from the A-delta and C fibers.

Any stimulation to the skin, including ultrasound, massage, heat, or ice can initiate this scenario. It is part of the reason pain can be altered by acupuncture and TENS—Transcutaneous **E**lectrical **N**erve **S**timulation—in which a pulsed electric current is delivered by a small battery-powered stimulator through thin wires to skin electrodes fixed to the area that hurts.

Once the electrical stimulation of pain reaches the spinal cord, it is routed to those areas that process the message by increasing amino acids and substance P (for peptide/pain). Contact is established with pathways to and from the brain that further moderate the pain sensation.

Other factors can influence the perception of pain. *Endorphins* (*endo* = endogenous, *orphin* = morphine), the body's natural analgesics, are secreted. *Serotonin* is a chemical messenger that the body uses to suppress pain. It also plays a role in depression, which is why antidepressants may ameliorate both depression and chronic pain. Studies have shown that tryptophan (an essential amino acid and serotonin precursor) added to a low protein, high complex carbohydrate diet can elevate the level of serotonin and increase pain tolerance.

Muscle spasm can either cause or result from pain as the body attempts to splint an injured part. Muscle relaxants such as cyclobenzaprine (Flexeril) or carisoprodol (Soma) are often prescribed. These medications affect the brain by occupying some of the receptor sites on nerve cells and blocking transmission of normal signals. As a result, fewer signals reach the spastic muscle, permitting it to relax (Figure 8-2). Another commonly used medicine is diazepam (Valium), which also has a direct effect on skeletal muscle.

A variety of diversionary techniques such as engaging in an intense conversation or watching a funny movie (vigorous laughing may actually mobilize endorphins) may serve to lessen tension and pain. *Biofeedback* is another procedure that is used for relaxation enhancement and pain control. Skin electrodes pick up muscle activity, which then is displayed by sight and/or sound. With this "feedback" the patient practices relaxing and pain control techniques to modify muscle tension.

Acupuncture is gaining acceptance as an alternative therapy in the practice of Western medicine. The placement of the superfine acupuncture needles, which is essentially painless, does not follow our anatomic concept of nerve distribution,

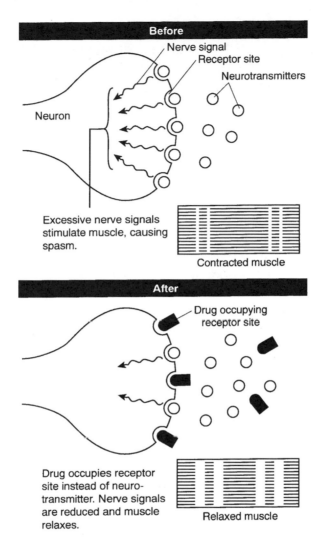

FIGURE 8-2   How muscle relaxants work.

Also, the concept of bodily energy—Qi or Chi—and its modulation has no counterpart in contemporary Western medical theory. Nonetheless, the insertion of the acupuncture needle activates the hypothalamus and pituitary gland, prompting the release of natural painkillers (endorphins) and antiinflammatory substances. The stimulation of the needle may also override and moderate other noxious stimuli in the central nervous system by "closing specific pain gates,"—this is the "counterirritation" mentioned earlier in this chapter.

Certain fragrances exert a calming effect and even lower blood pressure. Yale University has patented an apple spice fragrance because of its unusual ability to stop panic attacks in some people. Anxiety levels were also decreased by sniffing a perfume that contained essence of seaweed.

Music with a rhythm that approximates the resting heart (70 beats per minute) can actually slow a heart that is beating too fast. Some pieces are (1) *Venus, The Bringer of Peace (The Planets)* by Holst; (2) *Orchestral Suite #2 (Saraband)* by Bach; (3) *Mother Goose Suite,* First Movement, by Ravel; and (4) *The Brandenburg Concertos, #4,* Second Movement, by Bach. There also are a number of tapes specifically developed for this purpose. In contrast, music with an "anapestic" metre (two short beats followed by one long beat), which is the opposite of normal heart rhythm, can disturb the heart and initiate cardiac arrhythmias. Some acid rock music has been known to do this. The most familiar classical score in this category is *The Rite of Spring* by Stravinsky. "Smooth jazz" style Muzak (elevator background music) elevates the body's production of immunoglobulin A, a protective antibody.

TENDINITIS

Tendinitis is inflammation of a tendon. Swimmer's shoulder, jumper's knee, and tennis elbow are all examples of tendinitis caused by overuse. Treatment is to decrease inflammation through injections of antiinflammatory drugs such as a corticosteroid or medications such as nonsteroidal antiinflammatory drugs [NSAIDs, e.g., ibuprofen (Motrin), naproxen (Naprosyn)], icing, rest, and support.

Because improper athletic technique aggravated by poor sports mechanics or equipment and overtraining frequently results in tendinitis, such causes should be looked for and remedied. For example, breakaway bases could prevent as much as 71 percent of injuries in the 43 million Americans who play recreational baseball and softball. It takes 3,500 pounds of force to disassemble a stationary base, only one-fifth as much for the breakaway base. In 1995 emergency departments treated 13,000 children aged 5 to 14 for baseball injuries, 63 percent of which were caused by base contact. The use of the breakaway base could prevent 1.7 million injuries each year at a savings of $2 billion.

Tendons also can tear. The plantaris tendon, a vestigial structure in the calf, is frequently torn during sports such as tennis. A sudden painful snap is heard and felt in the calf. This is not a serious problem, requiring rest for only a brief period of time. A more critical condition occurs when the Achilles tendon tears. The appellation *tendo-Achillis* is taken from a Greek legend. Achilles, the son of Peleus and the Nereid Thetis and the hero of Homer's epic *The Iliad,* became the prototype of the Greeks' conception of manly valor and beauty. He was the most illustrious Greek warrior in the Trojan war and slew the Trojan hero, Hector. Achilles had been dipped in the River Styx by his mother. This rendered him invulnerable, except in the heel, where she held him when he was dunked and where he was fatally wounded by an arrow from the bow of Paris, Hector's younger brother.

The Achilles tendon is the strongest tendon in the body. It can bear up to seven times body weight without tearing. However, it can rupture when it is weakened and placed under undue stress. This occurs not only in the "weekend warrior" but also in the older person who, not noticing a curb, might take a misstep, coming down hard on his foot, bending the ankle up and forcefully straightening the knee in an attempt to keep his balance. When this occurs, the muscle–tendon complex is passively stretched at the same time that it is actively contracting, and it will give. The Achilles tendon can tear in a trained athlete or even in a ballet dancer such as Joffrey Ballet stars Gary Chryst and Gregory Huffman, both of whom suffered Achilles tendon tears while dancing. This significant injury may require surgery or at least prolonged cast immobilization for repair. The quadriceps muscle in the thigh can suffer a similar injury.

GAMEKEEPER'S THUMB

So-called "gamekeeper's thumb" is caused by stretching and tearing of the medial (ulnar) collateral ligament at the base of the thumb. English gamekeepers working on the royal estates were not paid very well. In order to provide fresh meat for their table, they often would poach for rabbits, dispatching them quickly by breaking their necks with a deft twist while holding the unfortunate animal firmly between the thumb and the index finger. Damage to the ligament was incurred in this fashion— hence the epithet. Nowadays this injury most commonly occurs while skiing by falling with the strap of the ski pole improperly wound around the thumb.

Although wrist sprains are not uncommon, a fracture of one of the small bones of the wrist can mimic a sprain. All wrist sprains should be treated as potential fractures—immobilized with a cast or a brace and x-rayed to rule out a broken bone.

FIBROMYALGIA

Muscle pain is the most common type of work-related injury and the second most common cause of visits to a physician. An estimated three million to six million Americans suffer from a syndrome called *fibromyalgia*. No one knows what causes it, and because it is so difficult to define, it is a called a *syndrome*—a collection of signs and symptoms appearing together—not a disease. Most of the patients are women and, in contrast to degenerative arthritis, it is prevalent among people in their mid-thirties and relatively uncommon in those older than 65. Fibromyalgia may begin in association with some type of muscle strain. Repetitive activities such as typing or computer keyboarding also may be responsible. Such "repetitive strain syndromes" result in significant loss of workdays and require vigorous treatment, including medications, splinting, and workplace modifications to limit mechanical strain while working. Sleep disturbance, stress from emotional or physical causes, immune system challenge, hormonal or chemical imbalance, weather change, or overexertion may act as triggers for attacks. Typically, discomfort is present on awakening and worsens throughout the day.

The term *fibromyalgia* means muscle and fibrous tissue (tendon and ligament) pain, which can radiate in characteristic patterns called referral zones. Insomnia, irritable bowel syndrome, morning stiffness, chronic headache, temporomandibular joint dysfunction syndrome, and fatigue are accompanying symptoms. Patients also complain of smooth muscle problems such as gastrointestinal (GI) cramping and diarrhea. All of these symptoms may present as episodes referred to as fibromyalgia storms or flares.

Chronic fatigue syndrome is another ill-defined entity that presents with some of the same symptoms as fibromyalgia and with chronic lethargy or fatigue. For years skeptical doctors wrote off patients' symptoms as psychological because medical tests were negative and the presenting complaints were accompanied by anxiety and depression. Even today some practitioners discount these diagnoses. But diagnosis can be difficult. Fibromyalgia symptoms, particularly pain and exhaustion, are a part of many diseases. Indeed, fibromyalgia often overlaps with other connective tissue disorders such as lupus. However, a knowledgeable physician can make a reasonable diagnosis by performing a "tender point examination." This examination is conducted by pressing on 18 specific sites located near the elbows, hips, knees, and neck, where the pain of fibromyalgia usually occurs. A diagnosis of fibromyalgia can be made if at least 11 of these points are sensitive, the patient has experienced pain for a minimum of three months, and the doctor has ruled out other causes for the pain. Dr. Alice Travell, the White House physician during the Kennedy Administration, first popularized the term *trigger-point* for these tender areas, which are thought to be painful because of ischemia (decreased blood supply), metabolic malfunction, or abnormal muscle activity that arises within muscle spindles.

Treatment is another problem. Patients need to find an understanding and believing doctor who is willing to patiently manage symptoms as they come and go. Regular stretching and exercise, such as swimming, walking, and other gentle activity, in spite of pain and stiffness, will help increase fitness and flexibility. Although not curative, heat and massage may provide significant symptomatic relief. Nonprescription analgesics and NSAIDs can be used to control pain. Commonly prescribed drugs include cyclobenzaprine (Flexeril), amitriptyline (Elavil), paroxetine (Paxil), doxepin (Sinequan), clonazepam (Klonopin), and alprazolam (Xanax). They increase the norepinephrine and serotonin neurotransmitters that modulate pain, the immune response, and sleep. Acupuncture and acupressure have also been used. Stress management through biofeedback and relaxation techniques may be helpful because muscle pain is aggravated by muscle tension resulting from emotional strain. Weight control and a well-balanced diet are advised, with the avoidance of nicotine and excess alcohol and caffeine.

There is no surefire cure for fibromyalgia because, to date, the cause has not been found. However, patients should be aware of bogus treatments such as unusual diets or special dietary supplements. So far there is no indication that fibromyalgia may be due to a deficiency of any vitamin or other nutriment.

Experts in rheumatology and arthritis often are knowledgeable about fibromyalgia. The Arthritis Foundation can serve as a valuable source of information for sufferers of this condition. You can write The Arthritis Foundation, P.O. BOX 7669, Atlanta, GA 30357-0669; 800-283-7800; http://www@arthritis.org. You can also get in touch with The National Chronic Fatigue Syndrome and Fibromyalgia Association, P.O. Box 18426, Kansas City, MO, 64133 (include a self-addressed, stamped envelope); 816-313-2000, for a 24-hour information line, or the National Institute of Arthritis and Musculoskeletal and Skin Diseases, National Institutes of Health, 1 AMS Circle, Bethesda, MD 20892-3675; 301-495-4484; 301-565-2966 (TTY for the hearing-impaired); http://www.NIH.GOV/NIAMS, or the Fibromyalgia Network, P.O. BOX 31750, Tucson, AZ 85751-1750 (800-853-2929; FAX 520-290-5550).

TORICOLLIS

Congenital torticollis (wry neck) is due to bleeding into the sternocleidomastoid muscle on one side of the neck with the formation of a hematoma (localized collection of blood, usually clotted) that organizes into scar tissue. This occurs sometime during the birth process. The back of the head is twisted to one shoulder with the chin pointing up and to the opposite side. The condition is progressive, and if it does not respond to stretching and/or an appropriate cast or brace, it may be necessary to relieve the contracture by bipolar (both ends) release of the offending muscle.

Other causes of a painful wry neck include direct irritation of the muscles themselves or of the cervical lymph nodes (lymphadenitis). The common garden-variety wry neck is of this type and often results from sleeping in a position that stresses the neck musculature or from exposing the neck directly to air conditioning for a prolonged period of time. This condition usually responds to moist heat, rest (which sometimes requires the use of a soft cervical collar), gentle massage, neck stretching, an antiinflammatory medication, and over-the-counter pain medications such as aspirin or acetaminophen (Tylenol).

Torticollis also may be associated with infection of the muscles or bones (osteomyelitis), injuries to the cervical spine, arthritis (both degenerative and rheumatoid), tuberculosis, contracture of scar tissue in the neck following a severe laceration or burn, scoliosis (curvature) of the cervical spine, meningitis, and ocular defects that require tilting the head to see properly. *Hysterical* torticollis is due to a psychogenic inability to control the muscles of the neck. *Spasmodic* torticollis, in which rhythmic convulsive spasms of the muscles of the neck occur, is the result of an organic disorder of the central nervous system. This condition currently is being treated with injections of botulinum toxin to temporarily relax the muscle.

A POTPOURRI OF MUSCLE INJURIES

Tears and Snaps

The biceps muscle in the upper arm is vulnerable to rupture, causing sudden pain. As a result of sudden indirect stretch in the aged, such ruptures may follow relatively minor trauma. The most characteristic physical finding is a convex bulge near the middle of the upper arm. Although there may be a cosmetic problem because of this, there seldom is enough weakness to warrant the extensive surgery necessary to repair the rupture. Three weeks in a sling accompanied by rehabilitative exercise is the customary treatment of choice.

"Snapping joints" usually are caused by slipping of a taut tendon over a bony prominence. Although annoying, they seldom are disabling and are very difficult to treat surgically because, once anesthetized, the muscle relaxes and it is not easy to passively elicit the snapping and determine exactly what soft tissue to release.

Loss of Circulation

Volkmann's ischemic contracture is a disabling contracture of the fingers and wrist that was first described in 1875 by the German surgeon Richard von Volkmann. It is due to compromise of the blood supply to the forearm as a complication of injuries of the upper extremities, particularly fractures about the elbow joint. However, anything that compromises circulation can cause a Volkmann's contracture, including the injudicious use of a tourniquet during surgery. The muscles of the forearm necrose (die), harden, and contract. The joints present unsightly contracture deformities and the hand often becomes almost completely useless. Treatment involves reconstructive surgery, the results of which are at best a form of damage control.

Compartment Syndrome

Increased pressure in the muscular compartments of the lower leg, thigh, or forearm can occur following tissue damage, bleeding, or swelling after trauma. It sometimes can take 12 to 24 hours to develop. This is a medical emergency diagnosed by physical examination—which demonstrates painful tense swelling, decreased feeling and movement in the limb, and loss of pulse—and by measurement of intracompartmental pressure (normal is 30 mmHg or less). Compartment syndrome is treated by immediate surgical decompression.

Sprains and Bursitis

A sprain (stretching of a ligament) is managed much as a strain is managed. Conservative treatment with immobilization, icing, elevation, and the use of a nonsteroidal antiinflammatory medication with subsequent graded exercise rehabilitation usually suffices. Surgical repair may be required if a ligament is torn.

Muscles and tendons that glide over bony prominences require a buffer between them and the bone to permit smooth gliding. A fluid-filled sac called a *bursa* does just this. All joints have adjacent bursa (Figure 8-2). The knee alone has 14 of them, and a condition called *bursitis* results when one or several bursae are irritated and inflamed. Treatment is similar to that for other soft tissue injuries and may include aspiration of

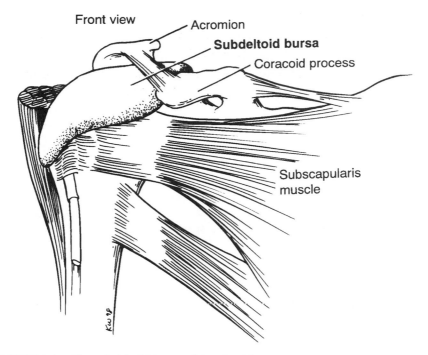

FIGURE 8-3 The subdeltoid bursa of the shoulder.

inflammatory fluid from the bursa and the injection of a corticosteroid to reduce inflammation.

Chronic or recurrent bursitis, such as that of the olecranon (tip of the elbow) or shoulder may require surgical excision of the offending bursal sac. "Housemaid's knee" is bursitis of the bursa overlying the kneecap, so termed because it occurred in housemaids who scrubbed floors while on their knees. Modern standup mopping and waxing techniques have made this condition all but extinct. "Weaver's bottom" is an occupational bursitis of the ischial bone found in weavers who sit on hard stools or cross-legged on a firm floor while weaving.

The *rotator cuff* is the tendon complex that supports the shoulder. Tears of this structure may result in chronic pain and an inability to lift the arm. It can be diagnosed by a special x-ray examination (arthrography) in which radiopaque dye injected into the shoulder is seen to leak out, or by an ultrasound or MRI study. Surgery for repair may be necessary; this often can be performed through an arthroscope.

SKATING INJURIES

Membership in the U.S. Figure Skating Association is more than 125,000 and growing rapidly. Skating injuries are not uncommon even in trained athletes. Almost half are related to overuse, most frequently involving problems with boot fit or the knee. Knee strain can occur with any activity that involves unusual stress applied to this joint. Treatment is along conventional lines—rest, ice, compression, and elevation followed by rehabilitative exercise. The quadriceps muscle typically is more developed in the landing leg in figure skaters. Pain at the inferior pole of the patella (jumper's knee) is not uncommon in these athletes. Local steroid injections or even surgical correction may be indicated. Stress fractures both in the legs and spine (spondylolysis) have been reported.

The major concern is soft tissue injuries of the foot and ankle related to poor fit of skating boots. Skating boots are heavy (an 8-year-old's pair of skates may weigh more than three pounds) and the boot is inflexible, compressing the soft tissues of the ankle between the upper portion of the boot and the bone. An excessively wide heel can cause the skater's heel to slip within the boot causing a "pump bump," a soft tissue bursal enlargement on the back of the heel. A combination last boot, which features a narrow heel and a broad forefoot, often will prevent heel slip. Padding of either the ankle or the foot, a small heel lift, or leather or synthetic foam shims help the heel fit snugly in the boot.

A very stiff boot is likely to cause boot-top injury, which can be anything from a bursitis to callus formation or tendinitis, and even a stress fracture of the fibula (outside leg bone below the knee). Padding should ameliorate this condition. Tenosynovitis of the tendons coursing over the anterior ankle can be caused by improper lacing. When laces are drawn too tightly, the top of the boot tongue compresses the ankle. To prevent this, the skater should make sure that the tongue is in a neutral position and that the skates are not laced too tightly. Bursal swelling over the malleoli (bony prominences at the sides of the ankle) is not uncommon. The leather of the skate boot can be stretched to avoid pressure, or a firm rubber doughnut can be placed around the bony prominence. Compression by the boot top can cause an

Achilles tendon injury with subsequent inflammation. Padding in the area of the boot counter is necessary. The boot should fit snugly at the heel to prevent sliding yet it must be large enough in the forefoot to accommodate toe motion. *Prevention* is the best way to handle boot-related problems.

TENNIS INJURIES

Tennis is a great way to enjoy activity with friends. It is also a vigorous sport that gets your muscles moving. However, you cannot just step from the office to the tennis court. Training is necessary to improve your health while playing your best game. A running program will enhance heart and lung conditioning. Workouts that consider all-around flexibility and strength are the best preparation for the tennis court. You can warm up with a brisk walk or an easy jog followed by stretching. Remember that warming up *means* getting warm. You do not have to feel pain, but you should sweat. Be sure to do lots of calf stretches because calf muscles become tight while playing tennis. This is especially true for women who spend time in high heels because their Achilles tendons tend to contract. Stay well hydrated during your match. Drink plenty of water but avoid alcohol, caffeine, and heavily sugared beverages.

Look to your shoes if you experience painful feet or legs. Sometimes an orthotic support is necessary. Running shoes are designed for forward motion, whereas tennis shoes are designed for on-court side-to-side moves. Select a shoe that gives you enough room in the toe and is well padded at the ball of the foot, where most pressure is exerted. The heel should also be padded for support. To avoid blisters, be sure your socks fit. Corns and calluses are pressure phenomena that indicate an underlying imbalance of the foot or a bony protuberance. They can be treated by moleskin padding. It is best to avoid commercial acid corn treatments.

Tennis elbow (lateral epicondylitis) is due to an incorrect backhand swing. Try a two-handed backhand grip, ice the elbow, use a tennis elbow strap just below the elbow, and get a lighter racquet (aluminum or carbon composite). Your racquet should be strung to approximately 50 pounds with a wide, well-padded handle to grasp. Take a lesson from a pro, and, if none of this works, see an orthopaedic surgeon for an examination, radiograph (to rule out calcification), and treatment (usually an NSAID or steroid injection, but sometimes surgery).

Tennis toe has the same etiology as turf toe. It is due to injury to the toes (most often the great toe) caused by sudden stops that cause pressure on the toenail. Bleeding under the nail occurs and is accompanied by severe, throbbing pain. The toe may swell and discolor. Treatment is with ice and painkillers. Padding and proper shoes can help prevent the problem.

AVOIDING INJURY

Injuries to soft tissues can be prevented by proper athletic training, including appropriate warming-up techniques. Overactivity is a setup for soft tissue injury, especially when it is of the "weekend type," and particularly when the athletic activity is age inappropriate. Stretching and strengthening through isometric exercising are good techniques to keep the amateur athlete fit and functioning. Our muscles want to serve us well and long, and they will if we follow a simple regimen to keep them healthy and avoid abusing them during activity.

A WORD ABOUT STEROIDS

Ever since Ben Johnson blew through the 100-meter dash at the 1988 Summer Olympic games in Seoul, Korea, running faster than any man in history, the problem of athletic steroid abuse has entered our national conscience. Johnson's feat was possible because he was using steroids. He subsequently was relieved of his gold medal. No chapter on muscle injury would be complete without considering the serious problem of steroid abuse.

Up to half a million high school students and hundreds of thousands of college students use steroids, at grave risk to their health. In fact, the abuse of steroids is one of the fastest growing drug problems facing young people today. One national study of college men showed that some are taking steroids simply to improve their appearance.

Steroids are psychologically addictive because men like the macho look they produce. Anyone who wants to gain 25 pounds for whatever reason can do so rather quickly with steroids. Steroids are a shortcut to building strength, and athletes know that they can increase their lean muscle mass by approximately 25 percent within about 10 weeks or so of training while using steroids. However, when you stop using steroids, your body returns to where it was before. So people take estrogen-blockers to prevent breast enlargement, downers such as marijuana and alcohol or tranquilizers to dampen their aggressive paranoia, and uppers such as amphetamines and stimulants as pick-me-ups. Their medicine cabinets begin to look like black-market pharmacies, and their health is on the way to being ruined.

Steroids do bring on dramatic muscle growth. The deltoids and quadriceps are unusually receptive to steroids. However, steroids are hormones and they greatly interfere with the body's normal hormonal balance. They can cause balding, personality disorders ("roid rage"), liver damage, elevated blood pressure and cholesterol, an increased bad lipoprotein (low-density lipoprotein, or LDL) level, suppression of white blood cells with a high risk of infection, and heart irregularities. It is a felony to sell steroids without a prescription, and it is a misdemeanor to possess them.

Some athletes buy steroids on the black market and use up to 30 to 60 times the recommended dosage prescribed for valid medical conditions. What is sold on the street often is phony or contains contaminants that are extremely harmful if swallowed or injected.

Insulin is another hormone that increasingly is being abused by bodybuilders in the false belief that it helps build muscle. In a nondiabetic person, too much insulin will deprive the brain of glucose and cause neurologic damage. The problem of misuse was so considerable in Great Britain in 1998 that the department of health made insulin available only by prescription.

Many athletes participating in sports that emphasize strength are taking oral creatine, an amino acid compound that is found naturally in skeletal muscle, heart, brain, and other tissues. Creatine supplements appear to enhance performance in short bursts of weight lifting and stationary cycling, but the data on swimming and running are not impressive. Side effects include renal dysfunction, GI disturbances, and muscle cramping. The long-term effect of creatine on the heart, brain, and other organs has yet to be determined.

But back to steroids.

Steroid use started in strength sports, such as weight lifting and bodybuilding, but its use quickly spread to football and other games in which aggressiveness and strength are important. Steroids are ideal for football players because they help build weight and strength and increase aggressiveness, which is exactly what you need to play well.

In adolescents, steroids produce severe facial and body acne as well as premature closure of the growth centers of long bones, which may result in short stature. In adult men, they can cause acne and an increase in aggressiveness and sexual appetite, sometimes resulting in criminal behavior and, after repeated dosing, impotence. Continued use leads to kidney damage, testicular shrinking, reduction of sperm production, enlargement of the breasts, and inflammation of the prostate. Additional side effects include jaundice and nosebleeds after a vigorous workout, symptomatic of high blood pressure. In women, steroids produce abnormal menstrual cycles and masculinization, including excessive hair growth on the face and body and deepening of the voice. Many of these changes can be permanent.

There are a few legitimate clinical indications for the use of steroids. Primarily they are prescribed for protein-wasting conditions such as severe burns. There also may be occasions for controlled use of steroids to treat certain cases of anemia, but generally the risks outweigh the benefits.

Junior high school students believe that they have to take steroids to play in high school, high school students think they have to take steroids to compete in college, and college athletes believe they have to take steroids to play in the professional leagues. It has been estimated that 50 percent of currently active NFL linemen use steroids.

Steroids are derived from the male hormone *testosterone,* which was isolated in 1935 and used during World War II to increase aggressiveness and muscle strength among German soldiers. Testosterone later was used to produce an anabolic (tissue-building) effect in burn patients and prison camp starvation victims. *Anabolic* steroids, in contrast to the corticosteroids (glucocorticoids) used in the treatment of some muscle diseases (e.g., polymyositis and dermatomyositis), first became popular among athletes in the 1950s, following reports of their use by Russian weight lifters at the Helsinki Olympics. Anabolic steroids enhance DNA replication and the subsequent increase in RNA and protein synthesis necessary for muscle growth. They recently were classified as controlled substances in many states, and they are prohibited by all amateur athletic–governing bodies. However, these drugs are still easily obtainable. Young athletes are using oral and/or injectable anabolic steroids, often in doses far exceeding both physiologic and pharmacologic norms. Usage is sometimes by a method called "stacking," in which increasingly larger doses are taken for a time and then discontinued for days or weeks before competition to avoid detection.

Among well-conditioned athletes who have trained to the point of a chronic *catabolic* (tissue breakdown) state, anabolic steroids increase strength and contribute to weight gain. The use of anabolic steroids and a high-protein diet does increase lean body mass and enhance performance. The increase in aggressiveness and euphoria seen in athletes using steroids enables them to train harder and for longer periods while taking the drug. However, the changes decrease with time, and steroid users require increasingly larger doses to produce continued results. Furthermore, the increase seen in size and strength is quickly lost when the drug is discontinued. Mark McGwire, batting star for the St. Louis Cardinals, came under fire during his 1998 season pursuit of Roger Maris's single-season home run record for using an over-the-counter testosterone-producing substance called *androstenedione,* which is banned by the National Football League and the NCAA.

The body's regulation of hormones is extremely delicate and is easily thrown off by any randomly added hormone. Increased vigilance and testing for the use of illicit drugs is necessary to eliminate their use. It is more important, however, that education in the risks of steroid use be included in programs on addictive drug abuse offered in our public schools—the earlier the better.

Injury is one thing, disease another, and unfortunately muscle is heir to many diseases, both hereditary and adventitious. The next chapter describes the most important of these diseases.

9

Diseases of Muscle

"A disease known is half cured."

Proverb

CLINICAL CLASSIFICATION

Disorders of muscle can be broadly classified into the *myopathies,* in which primary pathology is in the muscle itself, and the *neuropathies,* in which weakness is secondary to a disease of the nerve cell in the spinal column, such as poliomyelitis; the peripheral nerve, such as diabetic neuropathy; or the neuromuscular junction, as in myasthenia gravis. Further characterization is based on the genetics of these disorders when they are hereditary, their etiology (cause) when they are not, and the structural pathology of the tissues involved.

THE INVESTIGATION OF MUSCLE DISORDERS

The diagnosis of a muscle disorder is primarily a clinical problem. The history of its onset, its progression (including growth and development in a child), and the distribution of weakness or other symptoms is the mainstay of diagnosis. Establishing the presence of a similar disease in other family members points to a hereditary disorder.

Muscle disorders are common. They affect both sexes and all races. A careful history of a child's motor development gives important clues concerning what specific disease he may or may not have.

Many neuromuscular disorders are hereditary and most of these are *monogenic*—caused by the mutation of a single gene. Since the discovery of the location of the gene for Duchenne muscular dystrophy in 1985, 60 other mutations causing neuromuscular diseases have been detected as well as many more gene deletions and point mutations in the mitochondrial genome (special DNA for fabricating mitochondria, the muscle's energy "factories"). Therefore, a pedigree chart with a detailed family history is essential. Certain conditions are X-linked (carried by the female but passed only to the male). In *autosomal dominant* conditions, both males and females are in jeopardy, but only one parent need have the defective gene; this places 50 percent of his or her children at risk for inheriting the disease. In *autosomal recessive* conditions, both parents must have the defective gene for a child to develop the disease, and 25 percent of all children are in danger of inheriting it (Figure 9-1).

Clinical assessment requires a complete examination of the strength of various muscle groups and a comprehensive neurologic examination that includes measuring reflex tone and observing gait. Any muscle enlargement or atrophy is noted, and orthopaedic abnormalities, especially limitation of joint movement or scoliosis, are looked for.

Special tests include the measurement of serum enzymes. Creatine kinase (CK) is elevated in many diseases of muscle, but can rise in numerous other conditions, including heart attack, alcoholism, intramuscular injection, convulsions, meningitis, psychosis, acute abdominal crisis, hypothyroidism, pneumonia, eclampsia, radiotherapy, vigorous activity, and even sleep deprivation. Other chemical components of the blood can be assayed when tracking down specific diseases of metabolism that affect muscle. A variety of imaging techniques may help the clinician to make a diagnosis. Ultrasonography is a useful and practical method for screening muscle for pathologic change. Computerized tomography (CT) and magnetic resonance imaging (MRI) are valuable in the detection of pathologic change in muscle, particularly in deep muscles that are inaccessible to physical examination. Magnetic resonance spectroscopy (MRS) is a potent research tool in which the chemical components of muscle can be assessed.

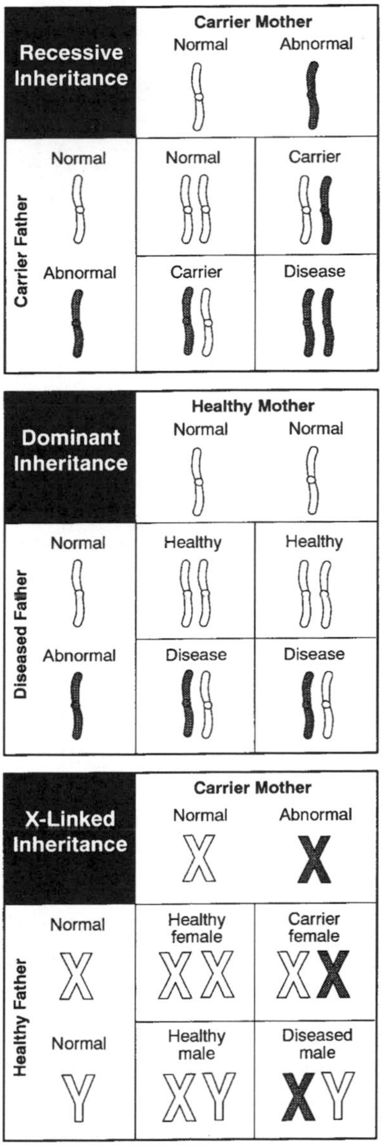

FIGURE 9-1   Patterns of inheritance.

Electrophysiologic examinations include the measurement of the conduction velocity of nerves, which is altered in certain diseases of nerve. Electromyography (EMG) is a valuable procedure used to visualize the electrical activity in muscle and to determine whether it is normal or abnormal and, if abnormal, whether it shows the characteristics of a neuropathic or myopathic process. The electrical pattern is observed on an oscilloscope, amplified, listened to, and recorded as a tracing. The readout is similar to that of an electrocardiogram.

A muscle biopsy taken with either a large-bore needle or through a small incision is easily accomplished without serious problem for the patient. It provides a specimen that can be stained for various constituents and analyzed with light microscopy, fluorescent techniques, or electron microscopy. Specific conditions show characteristic findings on biopsy. Nerve can be similarly examined.

MUSCLE DISEASE IN ANIMALS

Humans are not the only species susceptible to muscle disease. Some animals are also subject to these conditions.

Double muscling is a condition of farm animals, including sheep, cattle, and pigs, in which there is bilateral (both sides) enlargement of the muscles of the back, neck, and proximal limbs secondary to hyperplasia (enlargement). In cattle the condition is exploited for beef production in some local areas and breeds. As much as 20 percent more muscle can be present with essentially no fat.

A primary myopathy is found in Merino sheep. Stiffness of the legs results in a "rocking horse" gait because of inability to flex the hock and extend the stifle joints. This condition is progressive and may result in death from starvation. Some breeds of sheep are susceptible to a disease of glycogen storage. Glycogen cannot be metabolized for energy and accumulates in cardiac, smooth, and skeletal muscle cells. This is comparable to some glycogen storage problems in humans.

Murine muscular dystrophy is found in several strains of mice. This disease has findings similar in some ways to those of human Duchenne muscular dystrophy. Such dystrophic mice have been useful as an animal model for research into the cause and cure of Duchenne muscular dystrophy and other myopathies.

Muscular dystrophy of the mink is a progressive degeneration of skeletal muscle. Muscular dystrophy is rare in dogs but is found in golden retrievers and Irish setters. Such pedigreed animals are at higher risk for inheritance because of inbreeding.

Myotonia—increased muscle contractility—in goats represents the first known animal model of an inherited human skeletal muscle disorder. All myotonic goats are descended from a strain that first appeared around 1800 in central Tennessee. The condition is inherited as an *autosomal dominant* trait. There is no stiffness at birth but at approximately two weeks of age startling can provoke an attack during which the anxiety and initial movement to escape result in stiffness. The goat may fall to the ground and may even stop breathing momentarily.

Myotonia is also found in dogs, including chow chows and Labrador retrievers. A case of myotonia has also been reported in a horse and in Shropshire lambs.

Mitochondrial myopathies have been reported in dogs and sheep.

The *porcine stress syndrome* is a naturally occurring condition that can result in sudden death precipitated by stress. It is found especially in Landrace, Pietrain, and Poland China pigs.

Myasthenia gravis has been reported in both cats and dogs, and inherited chicken muscular dystrophy also has been seen. Ducks, turkeys, and even quail are prone to progressive myopathy. Mice carrying specific traits have been genetically engineered to provide animal models for the study of human disease. In addition to those mutated to study myopathy, a *transgenic* mouse has been bred that expresses the familial type of amyotrophic lateral sclerosis.

INFLAMMATORY AND INFECTIOUS MUSCLE DISEASES

Any tissue in the body, including muscle, can become inflamed or infected. Inflammation of muscle can occur as a manifestation of a systemic disease such as rheumatoid arthritis, systemic lupus erythematosus (SLE), or progressive systemic sclerosis. Other connective tissue disorders such as generalized inflammation of the blood vessels (polyarteritis nodosa or nodular myositis) or polymyalgia rheumatica also can produce myalgia and/or myopathy. *Sarcoidosis* may be accompanied by a granulomatous myositis. *Eosinophilic myositis* may include infiltration of muscle with eosinophils (a blood cell), which may cause a symptomatic myopathy whose presenting symptoms include muscle pain and tenderness. *Inclusion body myositis* is a chronic myopathy with slowly progressive weakness and wasting. It can be distinguished by the presence of typical *inclusion bodies* (round, oval, or irregular cellular structures) in muscle cells, which are apparent on electron microscopy.

A variety of viral infections can involve muscle. Everyone is familiar with the so-called "grippe" (from the French, "to seize"), a flulike disease that puts you to bed with severe muscular aches and pains. Acute myositis can occur with influenza A and B, adenovirus, coxsackievirus and echovirus, herpes simplex, or the Epstein-Barr virus. Epidemic pleurodynia, the coxsackievirus B5 infection, is characterized by severely painful trunk muscles. It occurs in outbreaks that affect children but not adults. Headache and fever accompany the muscle pain. In addition to wreaking havoc on the central nervous system, acquired immunodeficiency syndrome (AIDS) can cause a severe myositis.

FUNGAL AND BACTERIAL INFECTIONS

Fungal diseases of muscle also occur. Affected muscles are painful and the overlying skin may be involved. *Pyomyositis* consists of abscess formation in muscle. It is more common in the tropics and may be precipitated by a parasitic or viral infection, often with a history of trauma. The most common organism found is *Staphylococcus aureus,* but the streptococcus is seen in a small number of cases. The spread is through the blood. Management consists of surgical drainage and intravenous antibiotics. Any systemic fungus infection such as actinomycosis, coccidioidomycosis, sporotrichosis, or moniliasis, can affect muscle. The invasion of the bacteria *Clostridia botulinum* into devitalized muscle can cause gas gangrene.

TRICHINOSIS

The roundworm *Trichinella spiralis* is the parasite involved in *trichinosis.* Human infection occurs when raw or inadequately cooked pork (rarely, bear meat) containing encysted larvae is ingested. Live larvae eventually reach striated muscles, causing a myositis that is followed by calcification of the cyst wall of the larva. The diaphragm, pectoral (shoulder), and intercostal (between the ribs) muscles, as well as the tongue, are involved. The disease is distributed worldwide. Many cases remain asymptomatic. Close to 20 percent of the adult population in the United States is said to be infected. Muscle pain, swelling, and fever are cardinal signs of the inflammation. Various clinical disturbances may appear, including adenitis (inflammation of lymph glands), encephalitis (inflammation of the brain), meningitis (inflammation of the coverings of the brain and spinal cord), visual or auditory disorders, pneumonitis, pleurisy, or myocarditis (inflammation of the heart muscle). Treatment is with appropriate antibiotic therapy, but prevention is the best cure, and this includes consuming pork and pork products only when they have been well cooked.

POLYMYOSITIS AND DERMATOMYOSITIS

The prototype of a nonhereditary inflammatory disease of muscle is *polymyositis* (many-muscle inflammation). If a skin rash is present, the term *dermatomyositis* (skin-muscle inflammation) is used. Both these conditions can present acutely or run a subacute, relapsing, or chronic course. There are both childhood forms and adult forms. A bimodal age distribution has been reported, between ages 5 and 15 and then between 50 and 60 years. Polymyositis is as common as scleroderma, which involves a chronic shrinking and hardening of connective tissue, and half as common as systemic lupus erythematosus. Its incidence is 5 to 8 new cases per million people each year.

Polymyositis probably results from an autoimmune attack on the muscles by specialized immune system cells called *T cells*. The main autoimmune attack in dermatomyositis involves a group of proteins known as *complement* and *antibodies,* and there is early involvement of small blood vessels that supply muscles. Damage to muscle probably results from reduced blood supply rather than direct destruction of muscle tissue.

The cutting edge of research in the inflammatory myopathies is in understanding the immune system and autoimmune disease. The course and severity of the inflammatory myopathies vary widely in symptoms, progression, and complications. Weakness generally develops in a matter of weeks or months. As in multiple sclerosis, spontaneous remissions occasionally occur. Progressive weakness can lead to the need for use of a wheelchair or even bed confinement. Some physicians have found that the more rapid the onset, the better the chance of recovery. Approximately half of these patients improve with therapy. Without treatment, the inflammatory myopathies may lead to permanent disability or even death.

One function of the body's immune system is to produce specialized cells and proteins called *antibodies,* which fight infection. For reasons unknown, in autoimmune disease the patient becomes sensitized to his own antibodies, which then attack his own tissues. It is possible that some viral infections can trigger this autoimmune reaction. Although polymyositis and dermatomyositis are not considered to be hereditary diseases, the immune systems of certain people may be prone to autoimmune dysfunction. This trait can be inherited, but the diseases are not contagious.

Polymyositis is one of the few systemic muscle diseases in which pain is a cardinal symptom. Patients complain of aching and stiffness that is more marked in the arms, as well as weakness in the legs. However, approximately one-third present with a nonmuscular initial symptom. Associated findings include *dysphagia* (difficulty swallowing that can be due to pharyngeal or esophageal weakness or other eating difficulties) (Figure 9-2), dysarthria (difficulty in talking), and pain in the joints. Arthritis, usually in the hands, can occur in patients with chronic disease. Systemic symptoms such as fever, weight loss, and lethargy are common, and cardiac involvement has been reported.

Dermatomyositis is more severe than polymyositis. It appears to be more common in women, whereas polymyositis affects both sexes in approximately the same numbers. The presenting rash includes a butterfly-shaped violaceous discoloration on the face and a so-called heliotrope (color of the flower) rash of the eyelids. There may be swelling about the eyes and redness with a scaly rash around the face, shoulder, chest, back, elbows, or knees. Small papules are seen on the knuckles. Skin and subcutaneous calcification can occur late in the disease, mostly in children.

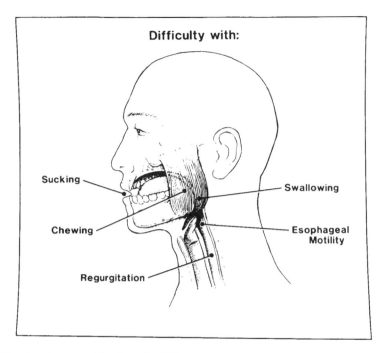

FIGURE 9-2   Causes of feeding disability.

Both dermatomyositis and polymyositis may complicate other connective tissue disorders (overlap syndrome) and may be found with rheumatoid arthritis, lupus, scleroderma, or periarteritis nodosa. Although the cause of inflammatory myositis is not known, all indications point to its being an autoimmune disease. As such, it is associated with an increased incidence of neoplasia (tumors). Dermatomyositis with onset after 40 years of age often is accompanied by a malignant disease, particularly in men. All types of malignancy occur, but carcinoma of the lung, breast, ovary, uterus, prostate, and stomach are the most frequent. In most instances, the manifestations of inflammatory myopathy precede those of the tumor, and treatment of the neoplasm may have a favorable effect on the associated muscle and skin lesions.

The childhood types of inflammatory myopathy usually are not associated with tumors. The skin lesions can be florid or minimal. The disease usually is of insidious onset, and presenting symptoms include severe malaise and listlessness.

Weakness in idiopathic polymyositis usually is more marked in the proximal upper limb than in the lower limb muscles, and the deltoids appear weaker than the hip flexors. The neck flexor muscles often are severely affected.

Elevation of the muscle enzyme creatine kinase (CK) may be very high, but it also may be nearly normal. Furthermore, CK falls during effective treatment or when the disease becomes inactive. CK levels are particularly useful in managing inflammatory myopathy because a rise in CK may precede an exacerbation of the disease by four to six weeks. *Erythrocyte sedimentation rate* (a blood test for inflammation) may be raised in about one-half of cases. The EMG shows a number of characteristic features in the acute stage, and muscle biopsy reveals inflammation of the muscle.

Systemic involvement includes joint pains *(arthralgias)* and calcium deposition *(calcinosis)* of subcutaneous tissue and the interstitial tissues of muscle. Hepatomegaly and splenomegaly—enlargement of the liver and spleen—can occur, as can pneumonitis with formation of fibrous tissue *(pulmonary fibrosis)* and gastrointestinal ulceration due to vascular inflammation. The heart and kidneys may be involved. Cellular death of blood vessels and other blood vessel pathologic *(angiopathic)* features are seen. Muscular contractures occur as weakness progresses.

Corticosteroids (as distinguished from anabolic steroids) are the mainstay in the treatment of polymyositis and dermatomyositis. They have acute side effects that include water retention, weight gain, hypertension, diabetes, and gastrointestinal hemorrhage. In addition, long-term complications include cataracts, infection and poor wound healing, psychoses, osteoporosis with fracture, delayed growth, and so-called *cushingoid* features [moon-shaped face, buffalo hump, central obesity, facial hairiness (hirsutism), and abdominal and thigh striations], as well as spontaneous tendon ruptures and acne with thinning of the skin. These serious side effects must be monitored. Adjuncts to steroid therapy include a low sodium–high potassium intake, antacids, and a high protein–low carbohydrate diet.

Immunosuppressant drugs also have been used, administered either alone or in combination with steroids. They usually are reserved for those patients who have not responded to steroid management. Such drugs include cyclophosphamide, azathioprine (Imuran), methotrexate, and cyclosporine (Sandimmune), as well as intravenous gamma globulin. These agents can be very toxic and cause bone marrow suppression, liver and renal toxicity, hypertension, loss of hair, and nausea and vomiting. Some may have a *teratogenic*—tumor-forming—effect. Plasma exchange (plasmapheresis), a technique in which antibodies that attack the muscle tissue are removed from the blood plasma, has been employed as an adjuvant to immuno-suppressive therapy. Plasmapheresis filters the blood by drawing it from a vein in the arm. A machine separates the blood cells from the plasma by centrifugation or filtering. The cells are then reconstituted in a plasma substitute and returned to the patient. The patient's plasma containing the aberrant antibodies is discarded.

Supportive measures include physical therapy to prevent or treat contractures, night splints as indicated, topical steroids for skin lesions, and diphosphonates for calcinosis in dermato-myositis.

The diagnosis and treatment of inflammatory myopathy is a challenge for practitioners. However, management can be gratifying because many of these cases respond to medical treatment.

ARTHROGRYPOSIS

Arthrogryposis (Greek: *arthro* = joint; *grypos* = curving) refers to a group of symptoms characterized by congenital rigidity of multiple deformed joints. It affects both sexes equally. Postural deformities most often involve distal joints such as the wrists, feet, and ankles (paradoxically there may be weakness of some muscle groups, even leading to dislocation of the hips); all are the result of immobility while still in the uterus. This may occur because of muscle paralysis resulting from a neuromuscular disorder or some other problem that limits fetal movement. Shortened muscles shrink and develop contractures. Joint rigidity can be lessened by manipulation and splinting, and surgical release of contracted soft tissues around joints should improve fixed deformity.

Not only can you have a myopathy in an isolated muscle or muscles (e.g., quadriceps myopathy), but you can also have an "isolated" contracture. This usually is due to multiple injections of an antibiotic or other medication and most often occurs where such injections are commonly given—in the shoulder (deltoid muscle) or thigh (quadriceps muscle). Along with congenital wry neck, congenital rigidity of the spine has been documented.

MOVEMENT DISORDERS

Involuntary movements can be seen in many diseases of the nervous system. *Dystonia musculorum deformans* is characterized by *dystonic* (abnormal tone) posture. Uncontrolled irregular movements can affect one or several limbs. Secondary deformities such as *foot equinus* (drop foot) can occur. An abnormality in a part of the brain called the basal ganglia is the culprit. Treatment of this condition is a problem. Muscle-relaxing drugs have been used but often are ineffective. Neurosurgical procedures that ablate portions of the brain are claimed by some to help. Tendon release and bracing have been helpful in selected patients.

Cerebral spastic palsy—or spasticity of one, several, or all four extremities—is due to an injury to the brain that results from endocrine imbalance, vitamin deficiency, or incompatibility of the Rh blood factor, which occurs when an Rh-negative mother gives birth to an Rh-positive child in her second or third pregnancy. Other causes include injury following hemorrhage due to trauma at birth, lack of oxygen because of winding of the umbilical cord around the baby's neck, oversedation of the mother, or aspiration of mucus by the child.

Any adverse incident that affects the brain after birth can cause *cerebral palsy* (CP), including trauma, infections (syphilis, meningitis, encephalitis), cerebral poliomyelitis, or vascular accident. The *antenatal* (before birth) type of CP is common in premature births. Newborns with CP who survive into infancy fall into three groups: those who are spastic, those who suffer from *ataxia*—loss of balance with incoordination, and those who show *athetosis*, which includes arrhythmic, purposeless writhing motions of the extremities. The stretch reflex is hyperreactive in spasticity, which produces orthopaedic deformities such as club foot *(talipes equinovarus)*, flexion of the knees, and a scissors gait or cross-leg progression accompanied by forward flexion of the hips.

Scoliosis may occur, and there are flexion deformities of the wrists, elbows, and shoulders. Mental deficiency may be present, but not necessarily.

Rehabilitation of the cerebral spastic patient requires intensive physical therapy, appropriate bracing, and surgery in selected cases. Surgery consists of tendon releases, lengthening, transplantation, division or partial excision of the motor nerves of spastic muscles, and selected operations on bone to improve stability and gait.

An unusual and interesting disorder is the so-called *stiff man syndrome.* Most reported cases have been men, usually in their fourth or fifth decade. Episodic stiffness occurs and becomes more persistent as the disease progresses. The face may be spared, but almost all other muscles are involved. The spine is tense, the abdominal muscles are tight, and rigidity may be absent during sleep. Medical treatment sometimes is effective.

A much less malign, more common, and troublesome problem is *restless legs syndrome,* which is found in adults and consists of unpleasant crawling or itching feelings experienced deeply in the thighs and legs. It seems impossible to find a position of comfort. Movement provides some relief—hence the appellation. Systemic causes should be ruled out, particularly *uremia* (an excess of nitrogenous waste in the blood), diabetes, peripheral neuropathy, and/or anemia. Using a foot cradle to keep the covers from forcing the ankles into plantar (downward) flexion may be helpful. Anemia and calcium imbalance are considered to be possible causes. Muscle relaxants and/or sedatives have been beneficial.

CRAMPS

Cramping in muscle involves a *hypercontraction* of muscle fibers. Often only a portion of the muscle is affected. Cramp is a common and usually benign symptom. It may occur in normal people after vigorous exercise, particularly when the body is not well conditioned. Residual stiffness and pain can be experienced for hours or days after a severe cramp, which indicates that the muscle was damaged by the cramp. Benign cramp is usually relieved by changing position and gently stretching the muscle.

Serious cramping can occur secondary to neurologic disease, certain metabolic diseases of muscle, and a variety of systemic disorders. These include chronic renal failure, tetany due to low calcium, depletion of salt, and hypothyroidism.

The management of cramp includes a workup to search for systemic metabolic factors, especially electrolyte (ionic) imbalance. Treatment is dictated by the underlying cause.

FATIGUE

Simple fatigue is well known to almost everyone. However, it also is the cardinal symptom of myasthenia gravis and occurs in diseases of the spinal cord such as amyotrophic lateral sclerosis (ALS, or Lou Gehrig's disease), of the peripheral nerves (e.g., hereditary neuropathy), or in diseases of muscle. When calcium is low for nutritional reasons, as in adult rickets (osteomalacia), muscle fiber excitation is disturbed and fatigue can ensue. Fatigue also occurs when many muscle fibers have been destroyed.

WEAKNESS

Weakness without medical cause may occur as a manifestation of a personality disorder or in people who are depressed or anxious. Such weakness shows rapid fluctuations and usually can be influenced by suggestion. No myotonia, wasting, or other objective findings accompany the weakness. Of course, a serious disease of muscle or nerve must be ruled out.

Cachexia (general weight loss and wasting) occurs during chronic infections, cancer, or malnutrition. It is due to protein catabolism (breakdown) within the muscle. The muscle usually recovers when proper nutrition is restored.

Loss of muscle occurs with aging. The force exerted by extending (lifting) the big toe is 30 percent less in those over 60 years of age than in younger people. Grip strength falls by almost half between 25 and 80 years of age. Unfortunately, these changes in muscular performance usually are accompanied by some impairment of fine touch sensibility, which can be measured by the ability to discriminate the pressure of two points in the fingers and vibration sense in the toes.

ALCOHOL

Myopathy can occur as the result of using many drugs. Most notable is alcohol, which may have either a direct toxic effect on muscle or an indirect influence because of fluid and electrolyte imbalance and malnutrition. Severe and permanent muscle damage can occur with chronic alcoholism. An interesting cause of muscular weakness is the ingestion of excessive amounts of licorice, which lowers the blood potassium necessary for muscular contraction. Alcohol does the same, as do certain purgatives and diuretics (water pills). In all of these, the weakness can be reversed by replacement of potassium. Many of the cytotoxic (cell-damaging) drugs used in the treatment of malignant disease can cause secondary myopathy.

ENDOCRINE DISORDERS

Many endocrine disorders have myopathy as an associated finding. The onset of weakness occurs slowly, with the muscles of the shoulders and hips being predominantly affected, and recovery usually occurs when the endocrine abnormality is corrected.

Muscular weakness is a common feature of *hyper*thyroidism. Muscles may become hypertrophied and muscular contraction and relaxation slowed in *hypo*thyroidism. Cramps and spasms can occur, and weakness occurs as the result of swelling of the muscles. Weakness in limb muscles associated with tenderness and aching occurs with the *osteomalacia* (softening of bones) found in hyperparathyroidism and other metabolic bone diseases.

Muscle weakness can be a complication of disorders of the adrenal gland (both hypo- and hyperadrenalism) as well as the administration of steroids for prolonged periods. Disorders of the pituitary can also affect the muscles. The muscles may be strong in the early stages of *acromegaly,* which involves enlargement of peripheral parts of the body due to an increase of growth hormone, but they become weak with fatigue as the disease progresses.

POLIO AND POST-POLIO SYNDROME

Poliomyelitis (infantile paralysis) is an acute viral infection that attacks the spinal cord, destroying the nerve cells that supply peripheral musculature. Acute paralytic poliomyelitis has long been a part of human history and has been documented since eighteenth dynasty Egypt (1580–1350 B.C.) There are an estimated 640,000 paralytic polio survivors in the United States, tens of thousands in Canada, and many thousands elsewhere in the world. In the past polio was a serious endemic and epidemic problem in the United States. The development of the Salk and Sabin vaccines has changed this; the last great polio epidemic was in 1952, the year the Salk vaccine was introduced.

Acute paralytic poliomyelitis is now uncommon in North America. Since 1965, after widespread vaccination, its annual incidence has been less than 0.01 per 100,000 in the United States. It has occurred as a rare complication of the Sabin live virus vaccine. Polio cases in any great number are now only found in Third World countries in which widespread vaccination is not practiced. The World Health Organization is committed to eradicate poliomyelitis by the year 2000. An estimated 116,000 new cases were reported worldwide in 1990, but the number of new cases was only 6,241 in 1994. If everyone were vaccinated, polio likely would disappear, as did smallpox some years ago. Residual paralysis and deformity resulting from the flaccid (floppy) paralysis of various muscle groups in the polio patient continues to present a challenge to physiatrists and orthopaedic surgeons.

Approximately one-third of polio survivors will suffer the late onset of fatigue, new weakness, and wasting, on average 35 years after their initial infection. They are not "getting" polio again. What they have is *post-poliomyelitis syndrome* (post-polio muscular atrophy) due to overuse of weakened muscles that the nervous system temporarily reinnervated after the initial attack of polio. Even with a loss of 50 percent of the nerves supplying a muscle, the surviving nerves were able to sprout additional neurons to achieve reinnervation. Hypertrophy of muscle generated further recovery of muscular strength. The problem is that after 30 to 35 years, these new neurons (nerve fibers) begin to get tired and wear out, and the muscle starts to languish. The most frightening thing is that this can happen in seemingly fully recovered or even uninvolved muscles that, of course, were involved but not enough to initially produce weakness. The patient complains of new weakness, fatigue, and pain.

Because the polio virus targets the central nervous system—the brain and spinal cord—a clinical or subclinical (undiagnosed) encephalitis (inflammation of the brain) may accompany the initial infection. This can leave polio survivors with increased fatigability, a lowered threshold to pain, and decreased respiratory competence. Such damage may lead to problems with sleep, swallowing, and breathing, all of which put a person at more than average risk when subjected to general anesthesia. Everyone who has had poliomyelitis also can suffer from the mechanical and arthritic changes that occur from orthopaedic deformity, including contractures and leg length inequality.

Many survivors of polio have a "type A" personality. They tend to overcompensate for their disabilities and are vigorous overachievers. When faced with the challenge of new weakness, they assume that strenuous exercise will rebuild strength. After all, intense exercise is what was originally recommended for treatment of their polio. This, of course, is the wrong thing to do, and it can be severely counterproductive. Treatment of this syndrome consists of carefully supervised graded isometric exercise and a high-repetition, low-load, nonfatiguing strengthening program. Swimming and gentle water exercise are good because the body is essentially weightless in the water and therefore the muscles are under less strain. *Fibromyalgia*, which frequently is found in a post-polio clinic, can be treated by trigger-point injection and with pain-relieving medication. Pulmonary function must be evaluated to rule out respiratory dysfunction. Sleep and swallowing studies may be indicated.

Orthopaedic deformities are managed with bracing and/or the use of a walking aid such as a cane, crutches, or a walker. An orthopaedic operation occasionally may be necessary. Pain can be handled with a TENS (**T**ranscutaneous **E**lectrical **N**erve **S**timulator) unit. Several medications have been useful in decreasing fatigue, including pyridostigmine (Mestinon), which is prescribed in myasthenia gravis, the classic disease marked by fatigue. However, the most important treatment for post-polio syndrome is a changed lifestyle. This may necessitate regular rest periods, particularly during the early afternoon when people can hit a "polio wall." Patients are encouraged to lose weight when necessary. Reducing work hours, changing work to a less strenuous vocation, or even retiring is sometimes necessary. With appropriate, sensible management, patients can be kept comfortable and functional. Post-polio muscular atrophy need not be as severe as it originally was thought to be.

Ongoing information on polio and post-polio syndrome can be obtained by networking the Polio Connection of America, P.O. Box 182, Howard Beach, NY 11414 (718-835-5366)—http://wwws.ios.com:80/nw1066 or the International Polio Network, 4205 Lindell Boulevard, #110, St. Louis, MO 63108-2915 (314-534-0475; Fax: 314-539-507; E-mail: Gini-Intl @ MSN.com).

MUSCULAR DYSTROPHY

Many muscle-wasting diseases are caused by genetic defects that lead to an aberrant or absent muscle protein. Most of these proteins function to lend mechanical support to the muscle fiber, but some are active in the cell metabolism. Muscular dystrophy (muscle–faulty nutrition) refers to a group of genetic diseases characterized by progressive weakness due to degeneration of voluntary musculature. Cardiac and smooth muscle may also be affected in some types of muscular dystrophy, and a few forms also involve other organ systems.

Muscle-wasting diseases affect all ethnic groups and nationalities. There are no known national borders. Some of these conditions occur in infancy or childhood, others in adults. The muscular dystrophies affect an estimated 200,000 Americans, about two-thirds of whom are children. The major types are Duchenne, Becker, limb-girdle, facioscapulohumeral, congenital, myotonic, oculopharyngeal, Emery-Dreifuss, and distal muscular dystrophy. Duchenne, Becker, and Emery-Dreifuss muscular dystrophies are named after the doctors who first described them. Limb-girdle, facioscapulohumeral, distal, and oculopharyngeal muscular dystrophy describe the location of muscular involvement. Congenital muscular dystrophy refers to onset at birth of this group of diseases. *Myotonic* muscular dystrophy is unique in that muscles are not only weak but also have difficulty relaxing (*myo* = muscle, *tonic* = tone). These diseases all are caused by genetic defects. Duchenne and Becker dystrophies represent a single disease expressing a variation in severity. Although a family history usually is present, sporadic mutation can cause an isolated case without an antecedent history of inheritance. The genetic flaw results in an abnormality of protein production in the muscle cell. Of course, these genetic diseases are not contagious.

The diagnosis of a muscular dystrophy is made by taking a careful history and conducting a thorough examination of the patient. An EMG and/or nerve conduction velocity test may be useful. Biopsy may show a typical pattern and may even be used to look for metabolites in the cell, such as glucose, fat, or *dystrophin*—the missing, deficient, or abnormally formed protein in Duchenne and Becker muscular dystrophy. DNA testing of the patient's blood can reveal a deletion (absence) of a necessary gene. Blood enzyme tests, particularly for creatine kinase, the enzyme that catalyzes energy-producing chemical reactions in the muscle cell, should be elevated, indicating leakage of this enzyme from the cell.

Genetics

We each have 46 chromosomes or sets of genes (same as the mouse and the banana). Half are inherited from the mother, half from the father. Flawed genes can be inherited, although a mutation can be present for the first time in a newborn. Many diseases of muscle and nerve are genetic. Genes are found in every cell in the body. They are coded and held in the DNA, which is wound very tightly in the nucleus of the cell. The DNA in each cell is 6.6 feet long and the cell nucleus is less than 10 micrometers (one micrometer is one millionth of a meter) in diameter. If all of your DNA were laid end to end, it would stretch for 476,000 miles, reaching to the moon and back. Of your chromosomes, 44 (22 matched pairs called *autosomes)* are made up of identical gene sets. One chromosome of every matched pair is inherited from each of your parents. The remaining two chromosomes are the X and Y. They determine whether an individual is a male or a female. A male has an X chromosome inherited from his mother and a Y chromosome from his father. A female has two X chromosomes, one inherited from each parent. So you see, it was your father who determined your gender.

As noted earlier in this chapter, there are three main forms of inheritance through which muscular dystrophy can be passed from a parent to a child. These are autosomal dominant, autosomal recessive, and X-linked recessive.

❏ When only one parent passes on a defective gene, inheritance is by an autosomal dominant pattern. Offspring run a 50 percent risk of inheriting an autosomal dominant disease.

❏ When both parents pass on defective genes, the child can inherit a recessive disease. If only one gene in the pair is defective, the other being normal, the person becomes a carrier with minimal, if any, symptoms or signs of the disease. Children of parents who carry a gene for the same recessive disease run a 25 percent risk of inheritance.

❏ Defects on the X chromosome lead to X-linked disease. These disorders are passed by the female exclusively to the male. This is because males have only one X chromosome with no normal X chromosome in reserve. Every son born to a female carrier of an X-linked disease (such as hemophilia or Duchenne muscular dystrophy) runs a 50 percent risk of inheriting the abnormal gene, and each daughter has a 50 percent chance of becoming a carrier (Figure 9-3).

In addition to available tests for the muscular dystrophies, there also are genetic tests for the carrier state. Carriers of Becker and Duchenne muscular dystrophy sometimes can be identified in childhood by a high CK level. There also are blood tests that compare their DNA with that of an involved sibling. The identification of the specific genetic abnormality in the muscular dystrophies has led to better diagnostic testing and a more thorough understanding of the biological basis of these diseases. Although the specific gene and absent or defective protein has not been identified in all of the muscular dystrophies, the chromosomal location of many of them has been established. It is hoped

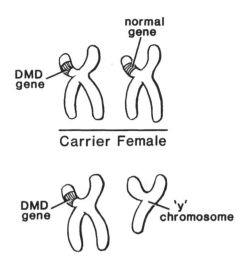

FIGURE 9-3   Patient and carrier chromosomes in Duchenne muscular dystrophy (DMD).

that such knowledge ultimately will lead to discovery of each gene and the protein it codes for, as well as specific therapies.

In the meantime, a medical program to maintain general health, surgery for the relief of severe contracture, bracing to keep the patient upright and mobile for as long as is feasible, and a variety of assistive and rehabilitative devices, including wheelchairs, reachers, canes, special clothing, and the like, can help the patient handle his tasks of daily living while functioning in a near-normal manner.

Respiratory management is available, including apparatus to assist breathing. Cardiac care and nutritional supervision are both important. Psychological and social problems must be addressed. Occupational therapy is used to assist the patient to meet the needs of his activities of daily living within the restrictions imposed by the disease. Physical therapy aids in augmenting and utilizing residual strength and relieving contractures through passive stretch.

As a general rule, the earlier clinical symptoms appear, the more rapid is progression of the disease. Genetic counseling is important. *Incurable* is not synonymous with *untreatable,* and proper treatment of the patient with muscle disease should be multidisciplinary and aggressive. In this way a patient can be helped to add life to his years and, in some cases, even years to his life.

The Muscular Dystrophy Association (MDA) is a voluntary health agency that provides comprehensive medical services through hospital-affiliated clinics and funds extensive research. Through its chapters, MDA offers diagnostic and treatment services as well as help with the purchase and repair of wheelchairs, braces, recreation at MDA summer camps, and selected transportation assistance. The association underwrites the diagnosis, treatment, and investigation of 40 neuromuscular disorders and conducts educational programs for the medical profession and the public. Funding is almost entirely through volunteer contributions. MDA's National Chairman is Jerry Lewis, who hosts a yearly Labor Day telethon to raise funds for the Association.

At an MDA clinic, a variety of health care professionals provide an interdisciplinary team approach to the management of neuromuscular diseases. For information on the Muscular Dystrophy Association and its programs and services, you can contact its national headquarters, 3300 East Sunrise Drive, Tucson, AZ 85718-3208, phone 520-529-2000 or 800-572-1717, or visit MDA's web site at www.MDAUSA.ORG.

The Types of Muscular Dystrophy

Duchenne Dystrophy

Duchenne muscular dystrophy is the most common childhood form of the disease. It is an X-linked disease, carried by the mother and affecting only her sons. Early signs occur at about age four years and include falling, difficulty getting up [children typically demonstrate a positive Gowers' (tripod) sign where they "climb up themselves" to rise from the floor] (Figure 9-4), difficulty ascending stairs, and a waddling broad-based gait due to symmetric weakness of the muscles of the shoulders, back, hips, and legs (Figure 9-5). As the disease progresses, there is an increase in lumbar lordosis (swayback) as the child tries to balance himself over his weakened legs. The calves are enlarged due to initial work hypertrophy (enlargement due to overuse) followed by degeneration and substitution of fat for muscle (Figure 9-6).

The defect in Duchenne muscular dystrophy is an absence of the muscle protein dystrophin, which contributes to the mechanical integrity of the muscle fiber. Structurally,

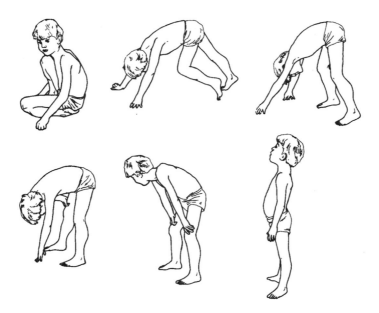

FIGURE 9-4   Gowers' (tripod) sign.

dystrophin resembles spectrin, an architectural component of the membrane of red blood cells. Although it represents only 0.002 percent of total muscle protein, its absence is devastating to muscular function. Mild mental retardation accompanies the disease in a small number of children. There are no

FIGURE 9-5   Distribution of muscle weakness in three major forms of muscular dystrophy: (A) Duchenne dystrophy, (B) limb-girdle dystrophy, and (C) facioscapulohumeral dystrophy.

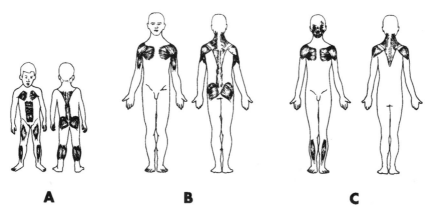

A   **B**   **C**

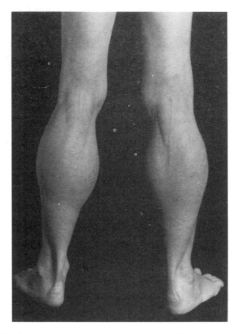

FIGURE 9-6   Calf enlargement in Duchenne muscular dystrophy.

abnormalities of sphincter control. Cardiomyopathy (muscular dystrophy of the heart muscle) occurs late in the course of Duchenne muscular dystrophy, as does respiratory difficulty. Selected patients can be kept standing and walking through the judicious use of contracture release, usually of tightened heel cords, accompanied by appropriate bracing (Figures 9-7 and 9-8). CK is markedly elevated early in the course of the disease but falls as less and less muscle becomes available for degradation.

Diagnosis is made on the basis of the typical history, hereditary pedigree, and clinical presentation; a gross elevation of CK with levels as high as 50 to 100 times normal, a typical pattern on EMG, DNA studies revealing an absence or abnormality of the dystrophin gene, and a muscle biopsy that shows characteristic histologic features as well as a lack of dystrophin by immunochemical staining.

With proper care, patients can remain upright and walking well into their teens, but a wheelchair eventually will become necessary. Once in the wheelchair, the child should be watched for the onset of scoliosis (spinal curvature), which may require

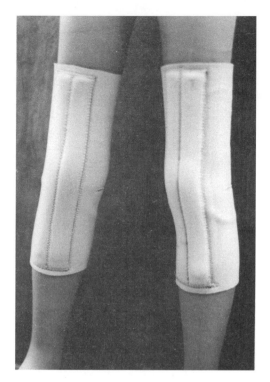

FIGURE 9-7   Neoprene knee sleeves with anterior spring-steel stays.

an external spinal containment support (brace or special seating) or an operation to arrest the curve (spinal fusion).

Carrier detection is part of the management of the family with a child with Duchenne muscular dystrophy. Female siblings should be screened for the carrier state. One way of doing this is with matching DNA analysis. Muscle dystrophin usually is normal in carriers, although some show mild signs of the disease such as calf enlargement or modest weakness. These "manifesting carriers" often have detectable abnormalities of dystrophin.

Duchenne muscular dystrophy occurs in 1 per 10,000 live male births, and its prevalence is 3 per 100,000 total population. This rather high mutation rate is due to the large size of the dystrophin gene. It is one of the largest human genes, comprising 0.1 percent of the total human genome, and thus presents a sizable target for mutation.

Corticosteroids temporarily retard muscle destruction in Duchenne muscular dystrophy. However, these drugs have

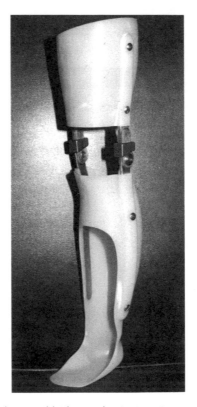

FIGURE 9-8   Tubular knee-ankle-foot orthosis (KAFO).

serious side effects, as described previously. Researchers currently are searching for similar medications with less toxicity.

There are several animal models of X-linked dystrophies, called Xp21 dystrophies because this is the location on the X chromosome where the gene causing muscular dystrophy is located. There is a mouse model, a dog model, and even a cat model. Using these animals (the dog seems closest to the human condition), recombinant DNA and molecular cloning technologies are being tested to explore the possibility of replacing abnormal genes in a patient's own cells. Problems include finding an appropriate *vector* (usually a virus) or mode of administration, restraining immune rejection, and exercising control of the gene once it is incorporated in the DNA of its host. Other areas of promising research include upgrading muscle metabolites such as *utropin,* which appears to supplant the absent dystrophin. The injection of normal myoblasts (immature muscle cells) directly into dystrophic muscles has so far been disappointing.

CASE REVIEW

Duchenne Muscular Dystrophy

Robert D. was the product of a normal full-term pregnancy. The family history was positive in that his first cousin, a son of his mother's sister, had a progressive debilitating neuromuscular disease. Robert did not kick much while carried in utero. His birth was normal but he walked late, complained of cramping in his legs on activity, and was considered a "clumsy child." Robert was of normal intelligence. He had increasing difficulty keeping up with other children during play. At age four, he was seen by a physician who diagnosed "flat feet" and special shoes were prescribed. Robert continued to show signs of increasing weakness. He fell frequently and had difficulty ascending stairs and jumping. When rising from a seated position, he "climbed up himself." He had no sphincter difficulty and no trouble breathing or swallowing. Although his walking gait was normal, he waddled when he ran.

At five years of age Robert was seen by a neurologist. His CK was 20,000 (over 100 times normal). Examination revealed symmetric weakness in his shoulders, hips, and knees. His deep tendon reflexes were depressed and his enlarged calves had a "rubbery" feel. He had modest contractures of his heel cords and tended to walk on his toes. There was no indication of the presence of an inflammatory myopathy. Electrical studies were not deemed necessary. DNA studies on Robert's blood failed to show a point mutation (deletion), and therefore a muscle biopsy was obtained, which revealed an almost complete lack of dystrophin. A diagnosis of Duchenne muscular dystrophy was made and the Duchenne pedigree was confirmed by correspondence with the physician who had made a similar diagnosis on Robert's cousin.

Because Robert was somewhat overweight and had difficulty controlling his appetite, it was decided not to place him on steroids for the time being, because they stimulate appetite. A physical therapist instructed Robert's parents in stretching exercises for his tight heel cords. An occupational therapist reviewed home and school activities that might help in his management. A dietitian provided a diet to reduce his weight. A social worker was consulted concerning his adjustment at home and in the community and contacted the school to inform them of the diagnosis and the fact that Robert would have difficulty managing stairs and required an adaptive physical education class.

If Robert can maintain his diet, he may be placed on steroids. In any case, he will continue to be seen on a regular basis. By the time he is 9 to 12 years of age, he might require tendon releases and bracing of his legs to continue standing and walking. A wheelchair may become necessary some time in his teens. A spinal fusion could be indicated if he develops scoliosis. Treatment of cardiac and respiratory complications will be available if needed.

Hopefully, research will develop therapies to arrest Robert's disease, thereby allowing him to recoup his strength.

Becker Dystrophy

The primary myopathies include Becker muscular dystrophy, which is similar to Duchenne muscular dystrophy in its appearance and distribution of weakness but considerably milder in its severity. Onset is later than Duchenne and patients are ambulatory into their third decade, with a longer life expectancy. Although dystrophin is present in Becker muscular dystrophy, it is decreased in quantity and may be abnormal in structure. Dystrophin mutations that disrupt the normal DNA reading frame (structural location) usually result in Duchenne dystrophy, whereas those that preserve the reading frame are more likely to cause Becker dystrophy.

Limb-Girdle Dystrophy

A third type of myopathy is limb-girdle muscular dystrophy, so named because the weakness mainly affects the shoulders and the pelvis. The range of severity in limb-girdle dystrophy is very wide. Although cases may be seen in childhood, the onset usually is in the second or third decade. CK is modestly elevated and progression of weakness usually—although not necessarily—is slow. Whereas Becker muscular dystrophy is X-linked in its inheritance, limb-girdle dystrophy is inherited through an autosomal recessive or dominant pattern. Molecular genetic studies have linked some forms of limb-girdle muscular dystrophy to abnormalities of specific proteins of the muscle membrane.

SCARMD

A number of these proteins form a complex, linking dystrophin to the muscle cell. Absence of or abnormalities in any of these so-called dystrophin-associated glycoproteins and dystrophin-associated proteins can cause a disease called **S**evere **C**hildhood **A**utosomal **R**ecessive **M**uscular **D**ystrophy (SCARMD). Symptoms, signs, and findings mimic Duchenne muscular dystrophy and account for what used to be considered an anomalous appearance of this disease in young girls.

Congenital Dystrophy

Congenital muscular dystrophy is the label applied to infants who show muscle weakness at birth and a dystrophic pattern on muscle biopsy. Such children are severely hypotonic (flaccid) but the disease usually is nonprogressive and therefore they should be treated vigorously to encourage functional use of available musculature. A number of congenital muscular dystrophies have associated central nervous system abnormalities. The prognosis is worse in these cases.

Emery-Dreifuss Dystrophy

Another X-linked muscular dystrophy clinically distinct from the Duchenne or Becker type is Emery-Dreifuss muscular dystrophy. This disease is characterized by mild weakness associated with widespread muscle contraction, including the back and elbows, and by cardiomyopathy (heart muscle disease).

Facioscapulohumeral Dystrophy

One form of muscular dystrophy predominantly affects the facial muscles and those of the shoulder girdle. This is called facioscapulohumeral muscular dystrophy (FSH) and its inheritance is autosomal dominant, although 10 percent to 33 percent of cases are sporadic (the defective gene is located on chromosome 4). The disease commonly presents in adolescence or early adult life. Cases that occur in childhood are more severe. There is a slow progression of weakness. In a fully developed case, the patient has a *myopathic* (flat, expressionless) facial expression and has trouble puffing the cheeks, sucking a straw, and wrinkling the forehead (some claim that Mona Lisa has such a face, her enigmatic transverse, dimpled smile resulting more from her heredity than from her state of mind) (Figure 9-9), difficulty in raising the arms for overhead tasks, severe "winging" of the scapulae (shoulder blades) (Figure 9-10), and ultimately some pelvic and leg weakness. Treatment is along conventional lines with bracing and various aids to facilitate chewing and swallowing. Prenatal testing is possible. An orthopaedic operation is available to stabilize a weakened shoulder.

Oculopharyngeal Dystrophy

An unusual myopathy common in French-Canadian families near Quebec and in Spanish-American families in the southwestern United States is oculopharyngeal (eye and throat) muscular dystrophy. This usually starts later in life with *ptosis* (drooping eyelids), facial weakness, and difficulty in swallowing. Other muscles may be involved later. Special eyeglass frames are available to prop up the eyelids; surgery can correct the drooping eyelids and the difficulty swallowing.

FIGURE 9-9   Mona Lisa.

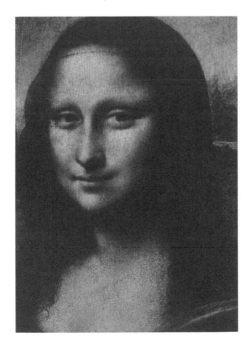

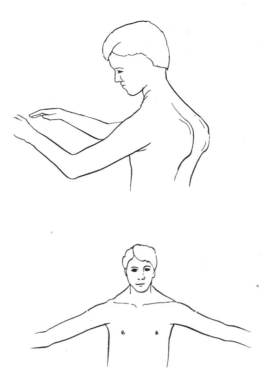

FIGURE 9-10   Scapular winging with shoulder weakness in FSH.

Distal Muscular Dystrophy

Distal muscular dystrophy describes a group of rare diseases in which the *distal* muscles—those of the forearms, hands, lower legs, and feet—are weakened. Difficulty in the grip and grasp is experienced. These dystrophies progress slowly and can be improved with supportive orthopaedic devices for the hands and feet.

SOME DISEASES OF MUSCLE THAT ARE NOT MUSCULAR DYSTROPHY

Floppy Infant Syndrome

The "floppy infant syndrome" is common in newborns. It is characterized by modest weakness with lack of muscle tone. Among its many causes is a group of muscular disorders referred to as the *benign congenital myopathies* of childhood and characterized by specific structural changes found on muscle biopsy. These myopathies of infancy are only slowly progressive and the pattern of inheritance is not clear. Muscle enzymes usually are normal, although the EMG is abnormal. Motor milestones often are delayed, and orthopaedic deformities such as elevated arches in the feet and scoliosis may be present. Such children have *dysmorphic* (badly formed) features that include a high-arched palate, an elongated face, a hollow chest, and long tapering fingers.

The structural changes of this group of "morphologically specific" myopathies seen on microscopy include central cores (central core disease), rods (nemaline rod myopathy), myotubes (myotubular-centronuclear myopathy), and disproportion of fiber type (congenital fiber type disproportion myopathy).

Metabolic Myopathy

The metabolic myopathies are a group of muscle diseases that occur as the result of biochemical defects of muscle metabolism. They vary in severity and may be progressive, fixed, or recurrent, with exercise-induced weakness, cramps, and sometimes myoglobin in the urine (myoglobinuria). There are nine known inborn errors of glycogen metabolism in which an enzyme deficiency leads to inability of the muscle to properly metabolize this source of energy. Attempts have been made to replace a missing enzyme and/or to treat some of these conditions with dietary therapy.

Myopathies due to abnormalities of lipid metabolism, resulting from mitochondrial metabolic defects, are characterized by neutral lipid accumulation in muscle. As with glycogen accumulation, abnormal stores of lipid are easily recognized by special staining on a muscle biopsy. Some of these conditions can be treated with replacement therapy, such as carnitine deficiency. Special diets are also beneficial. Other mitochondrial myopathies are diseases of the energy system of muscle and present an ongoing challenge to researchers looking for cause and cure. Current treatment consists of dietary manipulations and vitamin therapy.

Periodic Paralysis

One of nature's basic operations is the process of excitation through "voltage-gating"—transmission of an electric current through a molecular "gate." It has been conserved for more than

600 million years of evolution and brought to perfection in animals and human beings. The periodic paralyses are a group of muscle disorders characterized by attacks of paralysis with associated flaccidity. They occur as the result of disorders in the ion channels of the muscle in which, because of a voltage-gating disturbance, an ion such as sodium, potassium, or calcium has abnormal transit into or out of the muscle cell, hence the appellation "channelopathies."

These diseases tend to remit and relapse. Three distinct types have been described, depending on whether serum potassium (K) is high, normal, or low during the attack. Intervals between attacks may vary from days to weeks or months, and even years. In some cases their severity and frequency tends to decrease with age, and the attacks may even completely disappear, especially in women. Palsy may be triggered by strenuous exercise and exposure to cold, and accompanied by tingling in the extremities and generalized weakness. Too little carbohydrate in the diet as well as insulin level can affect some of these conditions. Inheritance is usually by an autosomal dominant pattern that involves one or more of the 44 nonsexual chromosomes. Attacks of hyperkalemic (high potassium) and hypokalemic (low potassium) periodic paralysis often can be treated by changes in dict. Medication to prevent attacks is available for some forms of the disease. Myotonia—an increase in muscle tone—may be seen in several of the periodic paralyses. This is part and parcel of the ion channel disorder that causes these conditions.

Prader-Willi Syndrome

The Prader-Willi syndrome is known as the H3O syndrome, and involves Hypotonia (decreased tone, weakness), Hypomentia (low intelligence), Hypogonadism (underdeveloped sex glands), and Obesity. An abnormality at chromosome XV has been demonstrated in several cases. Patients have a typical appearance of fair hair, blue eyes, a high forehead, and small almond-shaped eyes. Diabetes develops in adolescence. There is marked hypotonia at birth. Compulsive eating begins in early childhood, leading to obesity accompanied by weakness, mental retardation, and a failure of the gonads to develop.

Malignant Hyperthermia

Malignant hyperthermia is a dramatic and often fatal condition initiated by a hypermetabolic state of skeletal muscle and characterized by a sudden and sustained temperature rise during general anesthesia (surgical stress). It is accompanied by rapid heart rate and breathing, muscular rigidity, and cyanosis (blueness of the skin). It occurs in 1:15,000 surgeries involving anesthesia in children; 1:50,000 in adults. Muscle is rapidly destroyed, with subsequent kidney shutdown. The condition usually is expressed as an autosomal dominant trait. Patients with a variety of myopathies, especially central core disease, are at risk for malignant hyperthermia. In suspected cases, a sophisticated test is available that requires a muscle biopsy. An attack can be aborted by the intravenous administration of the drug dantrolene sodium (Dantrium). Supportive measures include cooling the body and correcting the metabolic acidosis that occurs. Oral dantrolene sodium can also be given prophylactically before surgery. Renal status must be closely monitored after an episode of malignant hyperthermia.

Malignant hyperthermia is not the only anesthetic threat to the person with a neuromuscular disease. Anesthesia in these cases must be carefully monitored, preferably by an anesthesiologist who is familiar with the special problems posed by such patients. Anesthesia can aggravate preexisting cardiomyopathy and challenge compromised breathing. Certain muscle relaxants may cause a sharp rise in serum potassium, placing the patient at increased jeopardy for cardiac arrhythmia or arrest. Changes in body temperature and the dietary restrictions often associated with anesthesia and surgery are not well tolerated. The problems of dehydration and gastric dilatation during surgery demand attention. Needless to say, a modern recovery facility should be available for immediate postoperative care.

Myasthenia Gravis

Myasthenia gravis (MG) is an autoimmune disease of the neuromuscular junction that results from a reduction of available acetylcholine receptors at this site. It is characterized by fluctuating weakness and fatigability that improves with rest. This fatigability distinguishes myasthenia from the other myopathies. Relapses and remissions are common. MG is not contagious. It can be life threatening when muscle weakness interferes with respiration. Symptoms usually are restricted to the muscles of the eyes, muscles of swallowing, and the proximal limb muscles. Infantile, juvenile, adult, and drug-induced (d-penicillamine) types have been described.

Myasthenia gravis (loss of strength–severe) is said to be a disease of younger women and older men (Aristotle Onassis suffered from it). It can be diagnosed chemically by examining the blood for elevated acetylcholine receptor antibodies and with a special EMG that measures the electrical discharge of a single muscle fiber. Symptoms abate with a test dose of intramuscular or oral neostigmine or intravenous tensilon.

Myasthenia gravis is treated with anticholinesterase medications, commonly neostigmine (Prostigmin) or pyridostigmine (Mestinon). Corticosteroids are sometimes used, as are immunosuppressants such as azathioprine and cyclosporine or intravenous gamma globulin. Plasma exchange is available for a myasthenic crisis. Removal of the thymus gland (thymectomy) can lead to dramatic relief. This gland is part of the body's immune system. It is located in the chest behind the sternum and often is enlarged in patients with myasthenia gravis. *Thymomas* (tumors of the thymus) can be found in MG. They usually are benign.

Myasthenics must avoid nondepolarizing agents (drugs that interfere with the transmission of nerve impulses) because they exacerbate the disease. These include muscle relaxants; drugs that depress respiration, such as narcotics, barbiturates, and tranquilizers; and any drug that has a neuromuscular blocking action, such as the antibiotics streptomycin and neomycin.

There are congenital myasthenic syndromes as well as the Lambert-Eaton myasthenic syndrome of myasthenia that can be associated with cancer of the lung.

Myasthenia gravis usually can be managed medically. More effective therapies should be in the offing with continued research into this disease of the myoneural junction.

CASE REPORT

Myasthenia Gravis

Louis M. was a 61-year-old salesman who had always been in good health. He began to notice the slow onset of drooping of his eyelids followed by some shoulder and hip weakness and mild difficulty in swallowing. His symptoms were most severe in the evening and seemed to intensify in the summer and to be provoked by stress or repetitive tasks. He also was worse when he had a cold. Oddly enough, there were times when he was better, almost normal. As time went on, Louis began to detect a change in his voice and some difficulty in breathing.

Louis had diet-controlled diabetes. His mother was hypertensive and there was a positive family history of autoimmune disease.

Louis's doctor conducted an extensive workup to rule out lupus, rheumatoid disease, and thyroid conditions. An antinuclear antibody test was markedly positive and a CT scan of his mediastinum showed hyperplasia (enlargement) of his thymus. There was a marked increase in his acetylcholine receptor antibody level. He improved when given intravenous tensilon. A diagnosis of myasthenia gravis was made.

Louis is being managed with anticholinesterase drugs. If he does not respond, immunosuppressive therapy such as corticosteroids may be added. A workup to rule out associated malignant tumors was conducted and none were found. If his symptoms are uncontrolled with medical therapy, a thymectomy may be indicated.

MYOTONIC SYNDROMES

The myotonic syndromes are characterized by weakness accompanied by *myotonia*, a delayed relaxation or persistent contraction of skeletal muscle that can be elicited by tapping the ball of the thumb with a reflex hammer, inducing sustained contraction of this digit (Figure 9-11). Myotonia is also detectable on an EMG by its characteristic tracing and sound, much like a World War II dive bomber. As noted in the section on muscle disease in animals, a hereditary myotonia has been described in goats that is induced by

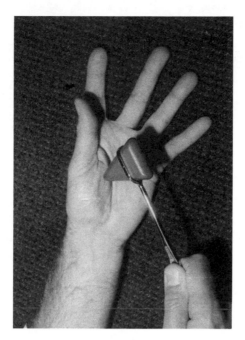

FIGURE 9-11   Percussion myotonia of thumb.

a sudden exertion or a loud noise. Such animals may freeze rigid in their tracks and keel over at the sound of the whistle of an oncoming train. *Springhalt*, a hereditary myotonic-like condition affecting horses, bears some resemblance to human myotonia.

Myotonia Congenita

The Danish physician A. J. T. Thomsen (1876) first described *myotonia congenita*, also known as Thomsen's disease, from his observations of the condition in four generations of his family. It could be traced back to his great-grandmother, whose family had emigrated to Denmark from North Germany in the eighteenth century. Thomsen was prompted to describe the disease because army medical officers refused to accept his medical certificate alleging his affected son was unfit for service in the Prussian army.

Patients with myotonia congenita have generalized muscular hypertrophy. They complain of muscular stiffness that is induced by movement and relieved by exercise. Myotonia may be aggravated by fatigue.

Paramyotonia Congenita

Paramyotonia congenita is a myotonic syndrome characterized by myotonia brought on or aggravated by cold. Symptoms usually are mild, and the condition especially affects the muscles of the hands and face. Weakness responds quickly to warming. As in myotonia congenita, there is a tendency to muscle hypertrophy. Muscle stiffness may be followed by flaccid weakness.

Myotonic Muscular Dystrophy

Myotonic muscular dystrophy, the most common muscular dystrophy found in adults, is an autosomal dominant multisystem disorder. Its most prevalent form usually becomes apparent in early adulthood, although the disease may present in childhood. It is characterized by myotonia, cataracts, gonadal atrophy, faulty carbohydrate tolerance, cardiac abnormalities, impaired pulmonary function that may present as "pickwickian syndrome" (from the description of the somnolent fat boy in Dickens's *Pickwick Papers*), hormonal dysfunction, progressive psychosocial deterioration, skull abnormalities, distal muscle weakness, and a typical facies that is long and lugubrious. The lids droop and the expression is thin and haggard. The temples are hollowed due to wasting of temporal musculature. Men suffer frontal baldness. Over three generations, dystrophia myotonica decimated the Royal House of Ypsilanti in Greece, for which Ypsilanti, Michigan is named. Myotonic dystrophy occurs because of a genetic fault on chromosome 19. The gene containing the flaw is for the enzyme myotonin protein kinase.

A variety of drugs are available to treat myotonia, including phenytoin (Dilantin), quinine (Quinamm), acetazolamide (Diamox), tocainide (Tonocard), and mexiletine (Mexitil). However, most patients are troubled more with progressive weakness than with the inability to release their grip. Their debility can only be treated with hand splints or leg braces. Cataracts can be removed, and the cardiac problems managed with drug therapy or a pacemaker if necessary. Labor and delivery may be complicated by muscle abnormality of the uterus.

Smooth muscle is affected in myotonic dystrophy. This often is expressed as difficulty in swallowing or abnormal bowel function.

Congenital Myotonic Dystrophy

The clinical manifestations of congenital myotonic dystrophy differ from those of the more common, adult-onset variety. Its main features are severe generalized floppiness at birth, with sucking and breathing difficulty. Such children are invariably born to mothers who have the adult form of the disease. *Hydramnios* (excess amniotic fluid) during pregnancy and premature delivery are common. Because the expression of myotonic dystrophy is highly variable, the mother herself may have few symptoms, the disease being diagnosed when she gives birth to a child with congenital myotonic dystrophy. These infants display a typical appearance, with facial diplegia (weakness), a characteristic tented mouth (shark-mouth), and an inability to fully shut the eyes (Figure 9-12). Such an expression has been seen on African masks (Figure 9-13). Severe clubfeet requiring early vigorous orthopaedic attention are present. Neither clinical nor electrical myotonia is demonstrable for a year or so. Mental retardation is a frequent feature of the disease. Affected children are at serious respiratory risk at birth. Should they survive, the more typical manifestations of adult myotonic dystrophy will develop with time.

FIGURE 9-12   Facies in congenital myotonic dystrophy showing tented mouth.

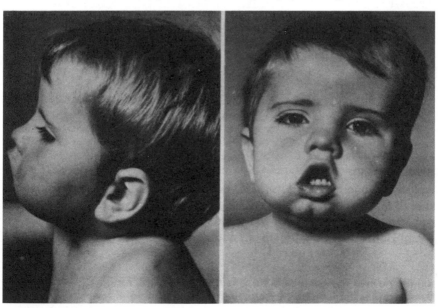

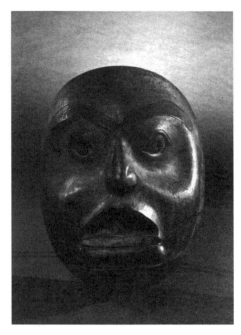

FIGURE 9-13   Primitive African mask with "tented mouth" of congenital myotonic dystrophy.

NEUROLOGIC DISORDERS THAT AFFECT MUSCLES

Spinal Muscular Dystrophy

Aran and Duchenne described spinal muscular atrophy (SMA) in adults in 1850. In the late nineteenth century the German doctors Werdnig and Hoffman characterized the condition in children. In the early 1950s Kugelberg and Weilander, two Swedish physicians, identified a juvenile form of SMA.

These subtypes comprise a group of inherited neuromuscular disease that affect the motor neurons that control the movement of voluntary muscle (see Chapter 5 for a discussion of nerve–muscle interaction). Degeneration of these cells in the brain and spinal cord prevents them from stimulating peripheral muscles, resulting in weakness and atrophy. The smooth muscle that controls bowel and bladder function as well as hearing and vision are not affected in SMA. The facial muscles are not seriously weakened, and the heart seldom is involved.

SMA is inherited as an autosomal recessive trait in which boys and girls are equally affected. The various forms are classified according to their time of onset, severity of involvement, and rate of progression. Most classifications include type I (severe), in which children are at respiratory risk at birth and never sit; type II (intermediate) is less severe, but the child never stands; type III has a later onset, and the child can stand alone and walk. Adult-onset SMA also has been described.

There also is a form of the disease known as X-linked spinal-bulbar muscular atrophy (Kennedy's disease). As the result of a defect in the androgen receptor gene on the X chromosome, affected males can have testicular atrophy, gynecomastia (enlarged breasts), and reduced fertility.

The presence of a family history of the condition greatly assists the diagnosis of SMA. Physical examination may reveal muscle *fasciculations* (irregular twitching), particularly in the tongue (a skinless muscle) and eyelids. A fine tremor may be present in the outstretched hands. Fasciculations sometimes are picked up on an electrocardiogram, which records muscle movement in the chest muscles overlying the heart. Muscle biopsy shows typical changes. EMG reveals a characteristic neuropathic pattern. CK may be normal or only slightly elevated. Intelligence is unaffected and indeed frequently is above normal.

The chromosomal location for the gene causing SMA has been identified. The location of the SMA gene is known. Further research in molecular genetics promises to isolate the gene and its protein product so that appropriate therapies can be developed. DNA studies may assist in making a diagnosis. Cells scraped from the inside of the cheek (fibroblasts) provide material for diagnostic testing. A carrier-detection test for SMA also is available.

Prognosis is very poor for SMA type I and unfavorable for type II. It is better in type III and the adult-onset forms of the disease. Treatment is supportive and symptomatic. It includes bracing to assist with standing and walking, appliances to facilitate the functions of daily living, respiratory support, and the management of scoliosis with electrical muscle stimulation, orthopaedic devices, and/or surgical spinal stabilization.

Families of SMA is a patient advocate group that raises money and circulates literature and information about the disease. Their national headquarters is P.O. Box 196, Libertyville, Illinois 60048-0196 (800-886-1762). MDA includes SMA among the neuromuscular conditions it supports, offering diagnosis and management in its clinics and underwriting worldwide research into the cause and treatment of the disease.

CASE REPORT

Spinal Muscular Atrophy

Susan C.'s parents were normal, and there was no family history of neuromuscular disease. However, she was always a weak child, somewhat floppy and with hyperextensible joints. On examination, Susan had a very fine tremor in her hands and atrophy along the edges of her tongue, which twitched (fasciculated). Her first six months or so of life were essentially normal and she was able to sit unaided. Her heart was normal and she had above normal intelligence. Susan could never stand. She had poor chest movement and breathed mostly with her diaphragm.

Susan was seen in consultation when her parents became aware of her weakness. A DNA examination of the cells scraped from the inside of her cheek revealed a diagnosis of spinal muscular atrophy. Susan's management was supportive and symptomatic. In addition, she was provided with a standing frame, and ultimately with a *reciprocating gait orthosis* (leg braces coupled to spring-loaded cables, which move them) and a wheeled walker so that she could move about her home. An electric wheelchair was provided for community mobility. She may require respiratory care as her disease progresses. Close contact with her school personnel is being maintained by a medical social worker.

With careful monitoring of her vital functions, particularly respiration, Susan can look forward to many years of productive living. Modern mobility systems such as the standing wheelchair, mobile breathing units, computers for study, and full-time aides, enable many people like Susan to attend college and enter the work force.

AMYOTROPHIC LATERAL SCLEROSIS

Lou Gehrig was the greatest first baseman in the history of baseball (Figure 9-14). He played in 2,136 consecutive games, a record broken only in 1995 by Cal Ripken Jr, the Baltimore shortstop. Lou Gehrig was known as "the iron horse" and had a lifetime batting average of .340. Only Babe Ruth hit more home runs during his career (714 to 493). Because of progressive weakness, he benched himself in May, 1939, and died in June, 1942, at the age of 38.

Gehrig died of amyotrophic lateral sclerosis (ALS), a fatal neurologic condition now also called Lou Gehrig's disease. It was first described by Charcot, the great French neurologist. *Amyotrophic* refers to muscle atrophy, *lateral* delineates that part of the spinal cord in which the nerve tracts affected by the disease are found, and *sclerosis* describes the dense scar tissue that remains after these nerves have degenerated.

FIGURE 9-14   Lou Gehrig (1904–1942).

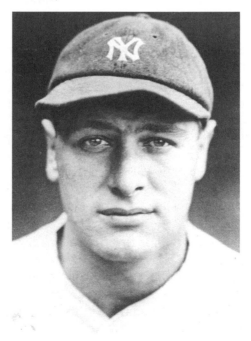

This rare disease affects approximately 1 in 10,000 people. There currently are about 30,000 cases in the United States, and approximately 5,000 new cases are diagnosed each year. Lou Gehrig was not the only notable person with ALS. Other famous people who have suffered from this condition include Henry Wallace (former U.S. vice president), Jacob Javits (former U.S. senator), David Niven (noted film actor), Steven Hawking (British physicist), Dimitri Shastokovich (classical composer), Ezzard Charles (heavyweight boxing champion), Dennis Day (radio and television entertainer), Matt Hazeltine (professional football player), and General Maxwell Taylor.

ALS usually affects adults, men more often than women. It may run a rapid (average 3 to 5 years) or slower (20 or more years) course. Approximately 10 percent of people who develop ALS have a familial history of the disorder. The inheritance pattern is autosomal dominant. A flawed gene on chromosome 21 has been identified. This gene codes for an enzyme that normally protects nerve cells against oxidative stress. It also has been suggested that naturally occurring substances in the body called *excitatory neurotransmitters* can damage motor neurons (nerves in the spinal cord responsible for movement). One of these, glutamate, is a prime suspect. A faulty immune system also may contribute to the nerve damage in ALS. Much research effort is being expended on investigating these possibilities.

The motor cells in the brain degenerate, causing spasticity, stiffness, and lack of reflexes. Axons from these cells run down the spinal cord in a pathway called the *corticospinal tract* and contact the anterior horn motor neurons that originate in front of the spinal cord. They cannot properly instruct these neurons, which in turn cannot function, resulting in a lack of muscle movement (paralysis). Muscles atrophy as these lower motor neurons die. As in spinal muscular atrophy, fasciculations occur, possibly due to spontaneous firing of the degenerating nerve cells. Although there is no specific test to diagnose ALS, EMG and nerve conduction velocity (NCV) studies are useful in assessing how well the nerves are working.

When lower motor neurons in the *bulbar* region (bottom of the brain) degenerate, the muscles responsible for swallowing, chewing, speaking, and breathing weaken. Some ALS patients lose emotional control, laughing and crying inappropriately. Involuntary muscles are not weakened, and the muscles controlling eye movement usually are not involved. Bowel and bladder function, hearing, touch sensation, vision, and intellect are unaffected. It has been said that ALS is a particularly cruel disease because it gives you a ringside seat to your own demise.

Treatment consists of antispasmodic drugs and medications to control cramping and salivation. Bracing and physical and occupational therapy are available. Respiratory support through ventilators can assist patients who have breathing difficulty. Foods that are easy to swallow aid digestion, and feeding gastrostomy (introducing a tube through the abdomen into the stomach) can provide nutrition when swallowing is no longer possible.

Several experimental medications are being studied, including riluzole and gabapentin, both of which block glutamate. To date, riluzole has been shown to extend the lives of people with ALS by about three months. Trials are in progress to study neurotrophic factors, natural substances that nourish nerve cells, and antioxidants, compounds that neutralize cell damage from oxidative stress. Some neurotrophic factors include brain-derived neurotrophic factor (BDNF), ciliary neurotrophic factors (CNTF), glial-derived neurotrophic factor (GDNF), and insulin-like growth factor I (myotrophin). Vitamins C and E, both potent antioxidants, are also under clinical trial. Some of these agents are administered orally, others by injection, and some by an abdominal "pump" connected through a catheter within the spinal canal.

Further information about ALS can be obtained through the Muscular Dystrophy Association or the Amyotrophic Lateral Sclerosis (ALS) Association, (818-340-7500; 800-782-4747 [patient hotline]).

CHARCOT-MARIE-TOOTH DISEASE (HEREDITARY MOTOR AND SENSORY NEUROPATHY)

Over 100 years ago, three physicians, Charcot and Marie of France and Tooth of England, described almost simultaneously the hereditary sensory and motor neuropathy that bears their names.

Charcot-Marie-Tooth (CMT) disease is a degenerative condition of the peripheral nerves, which have their cell bodies either in the brain or in the spinal cord. Voluntary muscle movement is primarily affected, although sensation, including pressure, pain, position and temperature, is also involved, although to a lesser degree.

About one of 2,500 people has Charcot-Marie-Tooth disease. It is one of the most common hereditary disorders, with a prevalence of 100,000 to 125,000 people in the United States. There are distinct forms of the disease, each caused by a separate genetic defect.

Approximately two-thirds of Charcot-Marie-Tooth patients have type I, which affects the myelin sheath, the fatty insulation that surrounds the nerves, much as insulation covers electrical wires. Myelin is the Greek word for "marrow." It was believed that white matter was the marrow of the brain, somewhat like the marrow of bone. Defects in this myelin covering cause nerve conduction to slow. About a third of patients have type II CMT, which affects the nerve fibers (axons) directly. A third type of this condition is known as Déjérine-Sottas disease, named after the two French doctors who first described it. This hypertrophic neuropathy of infancy is characterized by slow development of motor skills with severe sensory problems, hearing loss, and in some cases scoliosis requiring spinal fusion, and wheelchair confinement by the third or fourth decade.

Finally, Refsum's disease is distinguished by an excess of phytanic acid, a fatty acid metabolite, which leads to pigmentation of the retina, ataxia, hearing loss, and cardiac abnormalities. Severe foot deformities and scoliosis are present and early loss of the ability to walk is usual.

The myelin-related and axonal types of CMT show slow progression, which may not become apparent until late childhood or adolescence. The earliest symptoms usually are foot abnormalities such as high arches, twisting in of the foot from the ankle, and clawing of the toes (Figure 9-15). Wasting of the small muscles in the hands with subsequent deformity also can be present. Loss of sensation is seen. In the myelin-related type the nerves may become hypertrophic (enlarged) even though the extremity is wasted. This is due to swelling of the abnormal myelin. The speed of electrical transmission is markedly slowed

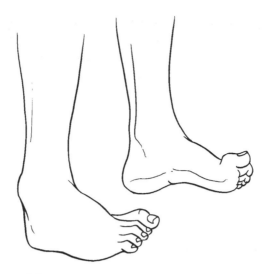

FIGURE 9-15   Foot deformity in CMT.

on the nerve conduction velocity test. In the "neuronal" (axonal) type of CMT, there is no nerve enlargement and the conduction velocity test is normal, but because less nerve stimulation is getting through the diseased nerve fiber, there is a decreased amplitude of the electric response seen on EMG.

CMT can be disabling, and splints, aids, or surgery to assist hand activity may be needed. Braces and corrective stabilizing operations are available for foot deformity. CMT does not affect the vital systems such as the heart and lungs. It is not contagious and life expectancy is not shortened.

The inheritance of Charcot-Marie-Tooth disease usually is autosomal dominant, in which a child need inherit an abnormal gene from only one parent to become symptomatic. In X-linked CMT, females may express the disease because this is an X-linked dominant condition, in which an abnormal X chromosome gene may come from either parent. Both males and females run a 50 percent risk of inheriting the defective X gene if the mother is the carrier. If it is the father who has the defect, all of his daughters will inherit the disease, but his sons will be spared because they receive a Y chromosome rather than an X chromosome from their father.

The defective genes of CMT have been found on chromosomes 1 and 17 and on the X chromosome. All of these affect myelin. The X chromosome gene also may affect the axon.

Future therapies will focus on influencing the molecular genetics of this disease and the other hereditary neuromuscular conditions.

The Charcot Marie Tooth Foundation provides information on the disease and ongoing research. Write CMT Association, Crozer Enterprise Center, 601 Upland Avenue, Upland, PA 19015 (215-499-7486). You may also contact MDA since it supports CMT clinical and research programs.

FRIEDREICH'S ATAXIA

Friedreich's ataxia was first described in the early 1860s by the German neurologist Nikolaus Friedreich. This inherited progressive disorder of the nervous system is marked by a gradual loss of motor coordination that expresses itself as unsteady movement (ataxia). The body fails to regulate its posture and coordinate its muscle movements, resulting in severe instability and loss of balance, which starts in the legs but eventually involves the arms.

Other motor symptoms include progressive weakness, scoliosis, and structural foot deformities. Decreased sensation also is a part of the clinical picture. The unsteadiness in the legs is aggravated by spasticity. The deep tendon reflexes are absent. *Dysmetria* (improper measuring of distance in muscular acts) occurs, vibration sense and lower extremity position sense are impaired, and nystagmus (rapid eye movement) appears. Walking is clumsy and poorly controlled.

Friedreich's ataxia is an autosomal recessive disease that can be seen in either sex. It usually appears between puberty and early adolescence, although it also can occur in early adulthood. Dysarthria (difficulty speaking) often develops. Cardiac disease is common, frequently seen as an abnormality in the heart's rhythm. Diabetes is found in about 30 percent of patients. Other associated defects include optic atrophy, cataract, deafness, abnormalities of the fingers, epilepsy, and mental deficiency.

The biochemical basis of this devastating condition is not known, but it is caused by one or several gene defects. Human beings have an estimated 100,000 genes. Whenever a genetic defect exists, proper protein (including enzyme) production for healthy cells is impaired. This can result in a disease such as Friedreich's ataxia.

Diagnosis is based on a positive family history and finding the typical picture on physical examination. EMG and NCV tests help rule out other conditions. Muscle biopsy is not particularly helpful. Nerve biopsy shows axonal degeneration. A test for the defective gene is available.

The major pathology is in the spinal cord, with both sensory and motor nerves affected, the cerebellum (the area of the brain concerned with coordination and balance), and other parts of the brain. The peripheral nerves also are affected.

Management is supportive and symptomatic. Although there is no cure for the disease, many of its symptoms can be relieved. Diabetes and cardiac problems are treated with medications. Braces and other orthopaedic appliances may prolong the ability to stand and walk. Corrective surgery for the feet and spine is available. Psychological counseling for the patient and family as well as genetic instruction contribute to a multidisciplinary management approach. In spite of this, most patients will require a wheelchair by the third decade and many die from cardiac complications before age 40.

Further information regarding Friedreich's ataxia can be obtained from the National Ataxia Foundation, 2600 Fernbrook Lane, Suite 119, Minneapolis, MN, phone 612-553-0020; E-mail NAF@MR.NET or MDA.

MISCELLANEOUS

There are other genetically determined and neuropathies that are acquired, such as inflammatory polyradiculoneuropathy (Guillain-Barré syndrome), neuropathies associated with metabolic diseases such as diabetes, vitamin deficiencies, renal and hepatic diseases; neuropathies due to drugs or toxic agents; neuropathies seen with malignant disease or infection; and finally, neuropathies accompanying connective tissue disorders.

TUMORS OF MUSCLE

Muscle neoplasms (new growth) are rare. Like all highly specialized cells, the muscle cell seldom undergoes neoplastic change. When it does, the resulting tumor can be highly malignant.

Primary tumors—those arising from the muscle itself—include the benign rhabdomyoma and the malignant rhabdomyosarcoma. The suffix *sarcoma* always indicates a malignant tumor from the mesenchymal layer of embryonic formation from which the muscles, connective tissue and bones develop. Rhabdomyoma is a rare tumor found in adults, most frequently men, that occurs in the chest, larynx, pharynx, and tongue. It also can be found in the heart in infants. Rhabdomyosarcoma is seen in childhood and mainly localized to the head and neck. It is a very aggressive malignant tumor.

Other nonneoplastic masses that occasionally are found in muscle include lipomas (fat), hemangiomas (blood vessels), myxomas (mesenchymal tissue), and fibromas (fibrous tissue). Local invasion by adjacent cancer can also occur. A metastasis to muscle is seen less often.

Destruction of muscle tissue from whatever cause or injury (such as rupture of a tendon), inflammation, or infection may produce a localized mass in the involved muscle that can be mistaken for a tumor.

This concludes our litany of diseases of nerve and muscle. Although most of these tragically disabling diseases lack a specific cure, there is an exceptionally active ongoing worldwide research effort searching for specific therapies, particularly in the field of molecular genetics. In the meantime, through a program of thoughtful care, the frustrating aspects of these conditions can be minimized while maximizing the benefits obtained through available treatment, increasing comfort and function, and enabling the patient to live as fully as possible for as long as is feasible.

10

Research

"Nothing is so difficult but that it may be found out by seeking."

Terence (185–159 B.C.)

Since the discovery of the dystrophin gene in 1986, scientists have been actively engaged in gene therapy research in an effort to develop a genetically engineered treatment for Duchenne muscular dystrophy (DMD). Three major obstacles hamper this line of research. First, the dystrophin gene is extremely large—some 200 times larger than most others. Its size prevents delivery to the muscle cell by most viral genes (vectors). The second problem is that large quantities of normal gene must be conveyed to muscles throughout the body. Finally, any virus used must be safe, without side effects, toxicity, or risk of rejection by the body's immune defenses.

To date, muscle genes have been isolated and used successfully in animal models. It is apparent that muscular dystrophy *can* be medically managed; it is only a question of *when* this will be accomplished. The dedicated and elegant work of investigators has resulted in the development of a highly altered version of an adenovirus (cold virus). All viral genes were removed from this cold virus, which opened up enough space to accommodate the dystrophin gene. In addition, removal of its viral genes prevents the virus from triggering an immune response once it gets into muscle. Other viral vectors are currently being investigated.

One is the adeno-associated virus, a small virus that does not cause any disease. Adeno-associated virus spreads well throughout muscle fibers, inserting the gene with stability. It does not evoke an immune response and persists in expressing the inserted gene for a long time. Similar results with this virus have been documented in neurons. It also has been shown that DNA alone ("naked DNA"), with nearby blood vessels tied off, can be injected under pressure into muscle fibers, where it remains and functions. A technique to temporarily alter blood vessels to allow controlled egress of viral particles to be taken up by the muscles is currently under investigation. These methods open up the possibility of intraarterial delivery of genes.

As of this writing, a phase 1 trial (to determine safety) of a gene therapy construct in the sarcoglycan-deficient forms of limb-girdle muscular dystrophy has been approved by the U.S. Food and Drug Administration. A sarcoglycan gene will be injected into a foot muscle using an adeno-associated viral vector. The success of this research program will have implications for the treatment of other types of muscular dystrophy, indeed for the management of any neuromuscular disease whose origin lies in a defect of the genetic material.

Other lines of investigation include increasing the synthesis or "upregulation" of other possible compensatory proteins when the protein dystrophin is deficient. One such protein is the muscle protein utrophin, which normally is located at the neuromuscular junction. New molecular technologies are taking a long hard look at this possibility. Although "gene therapy" usually means adding a gene, other "genetic" strategies on the horizon involve changing the way a cell "reads" the genetic code. For example, the antibiotic gentamicin allows mice with DMD to make the protein dystrophin because it causes the cells to read through a DNA "stop signal." Yet another intriguing idea is the manipulation of *telomerase*, the cellular enzyme that controls growth, to grow muscle cells to replace those that are depleted in some forms of muscular dystrophy.

At the same time, aggressive therapy-oriented research continues to be conducted with new methods of treatment. Clinical trials of the steroid drugs prednisone and oxandrolone (in DMD), as well as the drug albuterol (in FHS), are ongoing. All three have shown promise in preserving muscle despite the presence of an underlying genetic abnormality. Drugs by design, rather than discovery, hold promise for future therapy.

Research in amyotrophic lateral sclerosis (ALS) has focused on substances known as neurotrophic (nerve-nourishing) factors and medicaments that increase the body's production of these metabolites, as well as inhibitors of glutamate, a central nervous system stimulator. Riluzole, a glutamate inhibitor, was developed through such research. Myotrophin, derived from neurotrophic factor IgF-1, is currently under investigation. ALS studies have been expedited through the use of a genetically engineered mouse that expresses disease similar to familial ALS.

Investigation seeking to answer the question of what goes wrong in the cells of people who have Friedreich's ataxia has discovered a buildup of iron in the mitochondria (energy-producing units) of the cells. Therapy may be developed based on this finding. Progress in understanding the operation of ion channels, the microscopic pores and cell membranes that permit passage of ions (charged particles) has led to a better comprehension of the pathology of the periodic paralyses and myotonic diseases. On the basis of this kind of research, the periodic paralyses are now being managed with dietary modifications and the drug dichlorphenamide.

Clostridium botulinum, a bacterium that produces the potent neurotoxin botulin, causes food poisoning and serious central nervous system symptoms that can lead to death by muscular paralysis. Refinement of this neurotoxin has provided a potent medication that can provide significant relief when injected under strict control into spastic muscles. Injections of this botulinum toxin (BoTox) has helped such conditions as spastic torticollis, focal dystonia, writer's cramp, and other conditions characterized by unremitting muscular spasticity.

While researchers are searching for cures to neuromuscular diseases, other workers have been developing new systems of bracing in an effort to keep patients standing and walking as long as possible. Some of these experimental braces stimulate muscular response, whereas others inhibit spasticity.

Special electrical stimulation of the muscles that control the spine in an effort to inhibit scoliosis is under study. Comfortable yet supportive wheelchair seating systems using newly discovered fabrication techniques also help in the management of the neuromuscular patient's spine. New bracing techniques using a cable-loaded mechanism can provide a reciprocating gait in patients who lack lower extremity strength.

A whole system of "myoelectric" braces has been used success-fully in getting wheelchair-using paraplegics up and walking. Some of these systems employ surface electrodes placed over the muscles and nerves of the legs, which, when stimulated, assist spinal cord injury patients to stand and ambulate with the help of a walker.

Other devices make it possible for some quadriplegics to per-form tasks with their arms that otherwise would be impossible, such as picking up a book or holding a pen. This is accomplished through the use of a neuroprosthetic device the size of a cardiac pacemaker that is surgically implanted with electrodes attached to hand and forearm muscles. Slight movements of the shoulder send electrical signals that cause muscular contraction, gener-ating greater strength than that available through a splint or even a tendon transfer. Miniaturization should allow more porta-bility with decreased cost for the device, which now costs approx-imately $60,000. Computer adaptations to assist augmentative communication are also available, as well as many equipment modifications to help a disabled person achieve functional inde-pendence in the home and community.

Veterinary research has discovered that mutations in a gene that normally curtails muscle growth can produce muscle-bound cattle. This gene encodes myostatin, one of a large family of proteins that regulate growth. Mutations in this gene have been found in the Belgian Blue strain of cattle, which develop up to 30 percent more muscle with lower fat when fed normally. Since this gene remains active in adult muscles, researchers are trying to determine whether inhibiting myostatin might benefit patients with muscular dystrophy or the muscle wasting often caused by AIDS or cancer.

Damaged heart muscle in rabbits has been shown to get a boost from skeletal muscle cells transplanted from their legs. This finding may lead to new therapies for patients suffering heart damage after a heart attack.

Many challenges remain, but as we learn more and more about all of these disorders of muscle metabolism, continued research will undoubtedly open doors to treatment and cure.

Suggested Readings

The Compass in Your Nose and Other Astonishing Facts About Humans, Marc McCutcheon, Jeremy P. Tarcher, Inc., Los Angeles, 1989.

A Book of Curiosities, compiled and edited by Roberta Kramer, Jonathan David Publishers, Inc., Middle Village, New York, 1990.

The Body, Anthony Smith, Penguin Books, 1970.

Save Your Knees, James M. Fox, M.D., and Rick McGuire, M.D., Dell Publishing, 1988.

Late Effects of Poliomyelitis, edited by L. S. Halstead and D. O. Wiechers, Symposia Foundation, Miami, Florida, 1985.

Biomarkers, W. Evans, Ph.D., and I. H. Rosenberg, M.D., Simon and Schuster, New York, London, 1991.

Muscles, Masses and Motion, E. Geoffrey Walsh, distributed by Oxford, Blackwell Scientific Publications, Ltd., New York, Cambridge University Press, 1992.

Managing Pain before it Manages You, Margaret A. Caudill, M.D., Ph.D., The Guilford Press, New York, London, 1995.

Muscle Disorders in Childhood, (2nd edition) V. Dubowitz, M.D., W.B. Saunders Co., London, Philadelphia, 1995.

Neuromuscular Diseases, M. Swash and M. S. Schwartz, Springer-Verlag, Berlin, Heidelberg, New York, 1981.

Disorders of Voluntary Muscle, edited by Sir John Walton (5th edition), Churchill Livingstone, 1988.

Muscle and Its Diseases, I. M. Siegel, Yearbook Medical Publishers, Inc., Chicago, London, 1986.

Duchenne Muscular Dystrophy, Alan E. H. Emery, Oxford Medical Publications, 1987.

Elements of Medical Genetics, (5th edition), Alan E. H. Emery, Churchill Livingstone, Edinburgh, London, and New York, 1979.

Diagnosis and Management of Muscle Disease, A. P. Galdi, S.P. Medical and Scientific Books, New York, 1984.

Myopathies, Jaap Bethlem, J.P. Lippincott Co., Philadelphia and Toronto, 1980.

Muscular Dystrophy in Children: A Guide For Families, I. M. Siegel, Demos Medical Publishing Inc., New York, 1999.

The Clinical Management of Muscle Disease, I. M. Siegel, J.B. Lippincott Co., Philadelphia, 1977.

The History of a Genetic Disease: Duchenne Muscular Dystrophy or Meryon's Disease, A. E. H. Emery and M. L. H. Emery, Royal Society of Medicine Press, Ltd., London, 1995.

Evaluation and Treatment of Myopathies, R. Griggs, M.D., J. Mendell, M.D., R. Miller, M.D., F. A. Davis Co., Philadelphia, 1995.

All About Bone: An Owner's Manual, I. M. Siegel, M.D., Demos Medical Publishing Inc., New York, 1998.

The Cell—Life Science Library, Time-Life Books, New York, 1972.

Bones, Muscles and Joints—The American Medical Association Home Medical Library, Reader's Digest Association, Inc., New York, 1992.

Facts About Series (Spinal Muscular Atrophy, Friedreich's Ataxia, Charcot-Marie-Tooth Disease, Amyotrophic Lateral Sclerosis, Muscular Dystrophy, etc.). The Muscular Dystrophy Association, Tucson, Arizona.

The Resourceful Caregiver (helping family caregivers help themselves), by the National Family Caregivers Association, Mosby Lifeline (1996). Call 800-25-4177.

Guide to the Evaluation and Management of Neuromuscular Disease, John R. Bach, Hanley & Belfus, Inc., Philadelphia, 1994.

Myology (Basic and Clinic), 2nd edition, A. G. Engel, C. Franzini-Armstrong, McGraw-Hill, Inc., New York, 1994.

BOOKLETS AVAILABLE FROM MDA

"Everybody's Different, Nobody's Perfect" —written for the child with muscular dystrophy.

"Hey, I'm Here Too!"—written for normal siblings of the child with muscle disease.

"101 Hints to 'Help-With-Ease' for Patients with Neuromuscular Disease"—handy ways to facilitate tasks of daily living at home and in the community.

"A Teacher's Guide to Duchenne Muscular Dystrophy"—facts about muscular dystrophy for teachers and school personnel.

"Breathe Easy: Respiratory Care for Children with Muscular Dystrophy"

"Journey of Love"—a parent's guide to Duchenne muscular dystrophy. Excellent presentation of the basic science, physical and emotional needs, education, and the family. Extensive list of reading and resources.

"Quest"—bimonthly MUSCULAR DYSTROPHY magazine. Feature articles on neuromuscular disease. Covers current research.

Glossary

ABDUCT: To draw away from the midline of a limb or the body

ABIOTROPHY: Progressive loss of tissue vitality found in a degenerative hereditary disease

ACHILLES TENDON: Heel cord

ACTIN: A protein of the myofibril that, acting along with myosin particles, is responsible for the contraction and relaxation of muscle

ADDUCT: To draw toward the middle of a limb or the body

AEROBIC: Functioning in the presence of molecular oxygen

ANAEROBIC: Functioning in the absence of molecular oxygen

ANTIBODY: An immunoglobulin molecule that interacts only with the antigen that induces its synthesis or with antigen closely related to it

ANTIGEN: Any substance that, under appropriate conditions, will induce a specific immune response and react with the products of that response

ARTHRALGIA: Joint pain

ATROPHY: Wasting

BALANCE (vector): The force line (vector) produced on weight bearing that should keep the body upright

BECKER MUSCULAR DYSTROPHY: A primary X-linked myopathy due to decrease or abnormality of dystrophin. Clinical presentation is similar to that of Duchenne muscular dystrophy but onset usually is later and progress is slower.

BIARTICULAR (muscles): Muscles that span two joints, causing movement at each on contraction

BIOELECTRIC (response): The electrical response that is generated by muscle and nerve tissue

BIOKINETICS: From the Greek—of or for putting in motion. The science of movement of the body.

CARDIOMYOPATHY: Noninflammatory disease of the heart muscle

CARNITINE: A muscle metabolite required for the mitochondrial metabolism of fat for energy

CARRIER: A person who harbors a recessive gene and therefore does not usually manifest symptoms of the disease but can transmit the gene to offspring

CATARACT: From the Greek, *portcullis,* an iron grating barring passage (perhaps because an ocular opacity and a portcullis are both obstructions)—a partial or complete opacity of one or both eyes

CEREBELLUM: The posterior part of the brain that is concerned with the coordination of movement

CONGENITAL: Existing at, and usually before, birth

CONNECTIVE TISSUE: The tissue that binds and supports the various structures of the body

CREATINE KINASE: The enzyme that catalyzes the phosphorylation of creatine by ATP to form phosphocreatine

DAG: Dystrophin-associated glycoprotein—Membranous molecular protein construct associated with dystrophin

DEEP TENDON REFLEX: Involuntary contraction of a muscle after brief stretching caused by percussion of its tendon. Some deep tendon reflexes are the triceps reflex, biceps reflex, patellar reflex, and Achilles reflex.

DEPOLARIZATION: Reversal of the resting potential in an excitable cell membrane when stimulated. The membrane potential becomes positive with respect to the outside potential of the cell.

DISTAL MYOPATHY: A type of muscle disease in which the distal muscles (those of the hands and feet) are primarily involved. Certain other myopathies may have distal weakness as part of their presentation.

DOMINANT TRAIT: A genetic pedigree in which the defective gene is carried by one parent, who expresses the disease. Fifty percent of his or her offspring (irrespective of gender) are at risk for inheriting the disease.

DYSMORPHIC (features): Malformed

EATON-LAMBERT SYNDROME: A myasthenic syndrome associated with malignant tumor (particularly oat-cell carcinoma of the lung) and characterized by proximal muscle weakness, which improves with exercise, and decreased deep tendon reflexes. Extraocular muscle weakness and ptosis are rare.

ECCENTRIC CONTRACTION: Contraction of a muscle while it is lengthening

ELASTIC ELEMENTS: The part of a muscle that is not contractile (myosin or actin filaments). This includes the fibrous coverings within the muscle that converge to form the tendon.

ELECTRODIAGNOSIS: Refers generally to electrical techniques such as electromyography (EMG) and nerve conduction velocity (NCV) studies

EMERY-DREIFUSS MUSCULAR DYSTROPHY: An X-linked myopathy with insidious onset in childhood. Signature findings include severe contractures of the neck and spine. There is slow progression without loss of ambulation. By mid-adulthood, cardiac conduction defects occur, which can cause sudden death.

ENDOMYSIUM: Fibrous tissue that envelops individual muscle fibers

ENZYME: A protein catalyst that accelerates chemical reactions without itself being destroyed or altered

EPIMYSIUM: Deep fascia surrounding the anatomic muscle

ERYTHROCYTE SEDIMENTATION RATE (ESR): Rather non-specific blood test for inflammation

EQUINOCAVOVARUS: Clubfoot deformity of the foot and ankle

ESOPHAGUS: Swallowing pathway between pharynx (back of mouth) and stomach

EXCITATION CONTRACTION COUPLING: The process of electrical stimulation of muscle, with protein (myosin-actin) coupling and subsequent contraction

EXTEND: To straighten

FACIAL DIPLEGIA: Weakness of the facial muscles

FASCIA: Sheet of fibrous tissue that invests muscles or other organs

FASCICULATION: Brief muscle twitching, usually visible through the skin, representing spontaneous discharge of muscle fibers, seen in neurogenic muscle atrophy

FASCICULUS: Bundle of muscle fibers (pl. fasciculi)

FIBER: A single skeletal muscle cell

FLEX: To bend

FLOPPY INFANT SYNDROME: Hypotonia seen at birth. Can be present in a number of conditions, including congenital muscular dystrophy, morphologically specific myopathies, spinal muscular atrophy type I, brain and/or spinal cord damage or lesion, and so forth.

FOOT DROP: Weakness in the ability to dorsiflex (bring up) the foot at the ankle. This results in a "slapping" gait, dragging the foot and tripping on the toes.

FRIEDREICH'S ATAXIA: An autosomal recessive disease resulting from spinocerebellar degeneration and character-ized by peripheral neuropathy with spastic paraplegia, ataxia, foot and spinal deformity, ocular changes, and mental deficiency

GASTROCSOLEUS: The muscle complex of the gastrocnemius and the soleus, which comprise the major muscle bulk of the calf and activate the Achilles tendon

GLYCOGENOSIS: A disease of the storage of glycogen. Not to be confused with glycogenesis, which is the synthesis of glycogen (production of glucose)

GOWERS' SIGN: Inability to rise from the seated position without support by "climbing up" the legs, due to quadriceps muscle and hip extensor weakness resulting in inability to extend (straighten) these joints. Also called the "tripod" sign.

GUILLAIN-BARRÉ SYNDROME: Acute idiopathic polyneuritis resulting in paralysis. The condition may affect the respiratory center of the brain.

HEEL CORD: The tendon of the triceps surae muscle group, which is composed of the medial and lateral heads of the gastrocnemius and the soleus muscle. The "Achilles" tendon. The strongest tendon in the body; it plantarflexes the foot for toe-off during gait.

HEEL VARUS: Position of the heel when it is twisted in toward the midline of the body, as opposed to heel valgus, when the heel is twisted out, away from the midline of the body. Heel varus produces a high, long arch in the foot. Heel valgus flattens the arch.

HMSN: Hereditary motor and sensory neuropathy.

HYPERKALEMIC (periodic paralysis): A condition of paralysis accompanied by an elevated blood potassium level. Hypokalemic periodic paralysis, in which the level of blood potassium is lower than normal, as well as normokalemic paralysis also occur.

HYPERTROPHY: Enlargement of muscle such as occurs in the calves of children with Duchenne muscular dystrophy

HYPOTONIA: Reduction of muscle tone

IDIOPATHIC: Of unknown causation (from the Greek *idios* = private)

IG: Immunoglobulin. There are five classes, designated IgM, IgG, IgA, IgD, and IgE. Subclasses are designated by number (e.g., IgG-1). Immunoglobulins are structurally related glycoproteins that function as antibodies.

INBORN METABOLIC ERROR: Genetically determined biomechanical disorder in which an enzyme defect produces pathologic consequences at birth

INCLUSION BODY MYOSITIS: An adult myopathy characterized by progressive painless limb-girdle weakness and a normal or mildly elevated CK. Its signature finding is vacuoles lined with characteristic filaments when a muscle biopsy specimen is examined by electron microscopy. Although inclusion body myositis is regarded as an inflammatory myopathy, it is unresponsive to steroids or other immunosuppressive drugs.

ISOENZYMES (isozyme): Structurally related forms of an enzyme. Each isozyme has the same mechanism but different physical, chemical, or immunologic characteristics.

ISOKINETIC EXERCISE: Exercise in which constant muscle tension is maintained as muscles lengthen or shorten

ISOMETRIC EXERCISE: Exercise that is performed against resistance without change in muscle length

ISOTONIC EXERCISE: Exercise performed with shortening of muscle but without change in the force of muscle contraction

JOINT: An articulation between two or more bones of the skeleton that permits motion. Joints may be fibrous, cartilaginous, or synovial. Synovial joints are configured in different ways to provide a large variety of movements. Some synovial joints have a condyloid shape. Others are gliding, hinge, ball-and-socket, saddle, or pivot-shaped.

KINESIS: Stimulus-induced movement responsive to the intensity of the stimulus

KINESTHETIC: Related to the motion of the human body

KUGELBERG-WELANDER DISEASE: Late-onset spinal muscular atrophy

KYPHOSCOLIOSIS: Both backward and lateral curvature of the spine

LDH: Lactic dehydrogenase, a liver enzyme, elevated in some muscular dystrophies

LESION: Pathologic or traumatic discontinuity of tissue or loss of function of a part

LGD: Limb-girdle dystrophy. A dystrophinopathy (dystrophin pathology) in which dystrophin is present but decreased or altered. Clinical presentation is akin to Duchenne muscular dystrophy, but of later onset and slower progression. Inheritance may be autosomal recessive or dominant.

LORDOSIS: The anterior concavity of the curvature of the lumbar (and cervical) spine when viewed from the side. Synonyms include hollow-back, saddleback, and swayback. The opposite deformity is kyphosis.

LUGUBRIOUS FACIES: The mournful facial expression found in myotonic dystrophy

McARDLE'S DISEASE: Weakness and cramping on exercise with myoglobinuria (myoglobin in the urine, which produces a dark brown color) due to deficiency of phosphorylase, an enzyme necessary for energy metabolism

MACROGLOSSIA: Enlargement of the tongue that can be seen in Duchenne muscular dystrophy

METASTASIS: The transfer (usually via blood or lymph) of (tumor) cells to a place distant from the primary tumor or organ

MINIPOLYMYOCLONUS: Fine tremor of the fingers seen in spinal muscular atrophy

MITOCHONDRIAL MYOPATHY: Myopathy secondary to defect in mitochondrial metabolism

MORPHOLOGICALLY SPECIFIC MYOPATHY: Congenital myopathy named for a specific morphologic change found on microscopy. Some examples are central core disease, nemaline rod disease, and myotubular myopathy. These diseases have a similar clinical picture, which includes hypotonia after birth, slowly progressive generalized muscular weakness, normal CK, and dysmorphic skeletal features.

MOTOR END PLATE: The bulbous enlargement of the motor nerve at the neuromuscular junction. The motor end plate mediates motor activity by generating an action potential, which is then propagated into the muscle fiber.

MOTOR NEURON DISEASE: Amyotrophic lateral sclerosis

MYOBLAST: The stem cell of muscle that evolves into a mature muscle cell

MYOEDEMA: Swelling of muscle. Seen in hypothyroidism and other diseases

MYOGLOBIN: The oxygen-transporting protein pigment of muscle

MYOKYMIA: A benign condition characterized by brief contractions of groups of muscle fibers

MYOSITIS: Inflammation of muscle

MYOPATHY: Disease of muscle

MYOTONIA CONGENITA: Thomsen's disease; a congenital condition of muscular hypertrophy with stiffness and weakness, relieved by exercise

NECROSIS: Cell death

NEOPLASIA (neoplastic): Referring to tumor, new and/or abnormal growth

NCV (nerve conduction velocity): The velocity at which electrical current is conducted along nerve. Slowed in hereditary sensory and motor neuropathy type I and other demyelinating diseases

NORMOKALEMIC (periodic paralysis): Intermittent weakness in which the level of potassium in the blood is normal

NUCLEAR BAG AND CHAIN FIBERS: Specialized muscle fibers found in muscle spindles that act as mechanoreceptors in the muscles, regulating response to stretch

NYSTAGMUS: The involuntary, rhythmic, rapid movement of the eyeball in a vertical, horizontal, rotary, or mixed direction

OCCUPATIONAL THERAPY: The medical specialty that trains and assists patients at home and in the workplace to attend to the tasks of daily living

OCULOPHARYNGEAL MYOPATHY: A myopathy common in French-Canadian and Spanish-American families, regarded as a mitochondrial disease, and characterized by external ophthalmoplegia with dysphagia. Onset is in the third or fourth decade, and pedigree usually is autosomal dominant

ONION-BULB FORMATION: Nodular appearance of the myelin covering of nerves in demyelinating diseases

OPHTHALMOPLEGIA: Weakness of the eye muscles

ORTHOSES: Technical terminology for braces

OXYGEN DEBT: "Debt" created by lack of oxygen during vigorous exercise, repaid through metabolic processing

PATHOKINETICS: Abnormal patterns of movement

PECTUS CARINATUM: "Keeled breast," a deformity of the chest in which the sternum is prominent. Also called pigeon breast, keel (like the boat) chest, or chicken breast. The opposite is pectus excavatum (funnel chest). May be found in the morphologically specific myopathies.

PENIFORM: Shaped like a feather

PERIMYSIUM: Fibrous tissue that subdivides muscle fibers into fasciculi

PES CAVUS: Elevated long arch of the foot. Seen in Charcot-Marie-Tooth disease and other neuropathic conditions.

PHENYTOIN: Trade name Dilantin. Anticonvulsant medication used to decrease myotonia in myotonic dystrophy.

PICKWICKIAN SYNDROME: Uncontrolled somnolence. Named after a Dickensonian character.

PLASMAPHERESIS: The removal of plasma from the blood with retransfusion of the blood cells plus normal plasma back to the donor

POLYNEUROPATHY: Simultaneous neuropathy of several to many peripheral nerves. Also called multiple neuropathy.

POMPE'S DISEASE: A disease of glycogen storage

PRONE: Lying face downward

PROPRIOCEPTION: Perception of body position mediated by proprioceptor organs found in muscles and tendons

PTOSIS: Drooping of the upper eyelid

QUADRICEPS: The four-headed muscle at the front of the thigh that attaches to the patella (kneecap) and extends (straightens) the knee and flexes (bends) the hip

QUININE: Medicine used to relax muscle spasm

RECESSIVE TRAIT: Genetic trait incapable of expression unless the defective gene is carried by both parents; regardless of gender, their children are at 25 percent risk of inheriting the trait.

REFSUM'S DISEASE: Hereditary motor and sensory neuropathy type IV, which mimics Friedreich's ataxia and is characterized by a hypertrophic neuropathy with excess phytanic acid in the serum

REGENERATION: Attempt of diseased muscle to repair itself during cycle of degeneration–regeneration

RESPIRATION: Breathing

RESTING LENGTH (of muscle fiber): The ideal length at which maximum tension can be developed in a muscle

RETINITIS PIGMENTOSA: Pigmentation of the retina seen in neuromuscular diseases such as hereditary motor and sensory neuropathy type V and oculo-cranio-somatic neuromuscular disease

ROMBERG SIGN: Falling or swaying of the body when standing with the eyes closed and the feet held together; the result of loss of position sense seen in a variety of neurologic diseases.

ROUSSY-LEVY SYNDROME: Hereditary motor and sensory neuropathy type I associated with a fine tremor of the hands

SARCOLEMMA: Membrane covering a striated muscle fiber

SARCOMERE: The repeating contractile unit of a myofibril

SATELLITE CELL: Elongated cells closely associated with a muscle fiber. They play a role in regeneration.

SCALE EFFECT: First described by Galileo, it tells us that for every unit linear increase in a solid body, the surface area of the body increases by the square of the unit, its volume by the unit cubed. This explains why a person with even an inactive condition limiting his ultimate muscle mass may, although initially ambulatory, eventually lose the ability to walk with growth.

SCAPULAR WINGING: Protrusion of the shoulder blades due to muscle weakness in facioscapulohumeral muscular dystrophy. This deformity inhibits shoulder movement

SCARMD: **S**evere **c**hildhood **a**utosomal **r**ecessive **m**uscular **d**ystrophy—Duchenne-like muscular dystrophy found in either sex and due to a deficiency or abnormality of dystrophin-associated glycoprotein

SHARK MOUTH: Inverted V configuration of the upper lip seen in congenital myotonic dystrophy

SIMIAN HAND: Hand appearing like that of a monkey or ape. Due to wasting of thenar muscles secondary to a lesion of the median nerve. Seen in Charcot-Marie-Tooth disease.

SINGLE-FIBER EMG: Test of electrical activity of a single muscle fiber. Useful in diagnosis and research of certain neuromuscular conditions.

STELLATE CATARACT: Star-shaped opacity located under the surface of the lens. Found in myotonic dystrophy.

STIFF MAN SYNDROME: Sustained repetitive activity of muscle fibers affecting both sexes, usually in adult life

TACHYCARDIA: Rapid heartbeat

TACHYPNEA: Rapid respiration

TALIPES EQUINOVARUS: Clubfoot in which the foot is twisted down and in on the ankle

TENOSYNOVITIS: Inflammation of tendon and its sheath

TETANUS: Sustained muscular contraction

THYMOMA: A tumor (benign or malignant) of the thymus gland. Thymomas are found in a significant number of people with myasthenia gravis.

TONGUE FASCICULATIONS: Abnormal twitching of the tongue (a skinned muscle), usually accompanied by atrophy and found in neuropathic conditions such as spinal muscular atrophy and ALS.

TRICHINOSIS: Infection with Trichinae. The disease is attended by diarrhea, nausea, fever in the early stages, and later by pain, stiffness, muscle swelling, circumorbital edema, sweating, and insomnia

TROPOMYOSIN: A muscle protein inhibiting contraction unless its position is modified by troponin so that myosin molecules can make contact with actin

TROPONIN: Globular muscle proteins that inhibit contraction by blocking the interaction of actin and myosin. When combined with calcium, troponin modifies the position of tropomyosin so that the myosin–actin interaction can occur.

ULNAR NEURITIS: Irritation of the ulnar nerve causing weakness in the muscles supplied by the nerve and numbness and tingling in its sensory distribution. Can occur as a result of pressure on a wheelchair armrest.

UPPER MOTOR NEURON (also called a motoneuron): The upper motor neurons are those in the cerebral cortex that conduct impulses to the cerebral nerves or the spinal cord. Upper motor neuron signs include limb spasticity.

VASCULITIS: Inflammation of blood vessels

VECTORCARDIOGRAPHY: The measurement, transmitted by electrocardiographic leads, of the display (usually on an oscilloscope) of the direction and magnitude (vector) of the electromotive heart forces during a complete cardiac cycle

VERTEBRAL CANINIZATION: Increase in the relative height of the vertebral bodies, which may ultimately become square in shape, as in the quadruped, which is seen in children chronically bedridden for any cause, as well as in Duchenne muscular dystrophy and other selected myopathies

VITAL CAPACITY: Respiratory capacity

WADDLING GAIT: Ducklike ambulation seen in advancing Duchenne muscular dystrophy because of weakness of hip musculature

WEDGE OSTEOTOMY: Corrective orthopaedic operation in which wedges of bone are removed to produce a more normal shape or position of the foot or other body member

WORK HYPERTROPHY: Enlargement of muscles due to exercise. Seen in the calves of patients with Duchenne muscular dystrophy early in the disease.

X-LINKED: Hereditary pedigree in which the defective gene is on the X (sex) chromosome. Maternal transmission is exclusively to male offspring (50 percent risk). Females are at 50 percent jeopardy of being carriers.

XO GONADAL DYSGENESIS: Turner's syndrome. A genetic trait leading to female masculinization, which can express a disease that appears like Duchenne muscular dystrophy

Z-LINE: The line(s) delimiting a single sarcomere along the length of the myofibril. The distance from one Z-line to the next constitutes a sarcomere.

Index

Note: boldface numbers indicate illustrations